Fauda Kwang

Reno – Nov 1990

APHASIA, ALEXIA, AND AGRAPHIA

D. FRANK BENSON, MD

Director, Neurobehavioral Center
Boston Veterans Administration Medical Center
Professor, Neurology
Boston University School of Medicine
Boston, Massachusetts

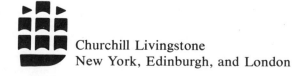

Churchill Livingstone
New York, Edinburgh, and London   1979

© Churchill Livingstone Inc.   1979

All rights reserved. No part of this publication may be reproduced, stored in a retrieval system, or transmitted in any form or by any means, electronic, mechanical, photocopying, recording or otherwise, without prior permission of the publishers (Churchill Livingstone Inc., 19 West 44th Street, New York, N.Y. 10036).

Distributed in the United Kingdom by Churchill Livingstone, Robert Stevenson House, 1–3 Baxter's Place, Leith Walk, Edinburgh EH1 3AF and by associated companies, branches and representatives throughout the world.

First published 1979

Printed in USA

ISBN 0 443 08041 0

7 6 5 4

Library of Congress Cataloging in Publication Data

Benson, David Frank, 1928–
      Aphasia, alexia, and agraphia.

      (Clinical neurology and neurosurgery monographs; v. 1)
      Bibliography: p.
      Includes index.
      1. Aphasia. 2. Alexia. 3. Agraphia. I. Title.
II. Series
RC 425.B46   616.8′55   79-17205
ISBN 0-443-08041-0

Foreword

With a great sense of the pragmatic as well as the theoretical implications for cerebral function, Frank Benson has written this eminently readable book. Aphasia, alexia, and agraphia, as disorders of symbolic language, are carried now conceptually well into the last quarter of the twentieth century. This is over a century from the beginnings of modern interest in these problems of brain dysfunction, especially in the halls of beginning French clinical neuroscience, then spreading into Germany and England. Always a challenge to physicians and scientists in related fields, these phenomena—particularly human, though lower animal communication does exist—have captured the interest and intellectual activity of many individuals concerned with man's most distinguishing brain function: language, its expression and comprehension, spoken, read and written. Interwoven themes of cerebral dominance, lateralization, anatomical features, developmental factors, physiological and pathological correlations have abounded, often dependent upon the investigator's conceptual bias. These works have produced a huge literature, critically reviewed by Dr. Benson.

Holistic versus the most minute brain localization theories form a background, with many considerations in. between, in wide-ranging variation. A veritable "Who's Who" in Neurology and associated fields of Psychology, Psychiatry and Linguistics have offered classifications. Many have felt that each person studying patients could and should develop his own methods and analysis of the language disorders. Certainly, historically, this is usually what has happened. A strong factor always has been the clinical-pathological correlation extant at a particular time, i.e., localized brain lesions due to wartime injuries, the focal lesions of cerebral vascular accidents and brain tumors. Parallel developments in the technology of clinical neuroscience have been most useful, especially cerebral air encephalography, arteriography, blood flow measurements, electroencephalography and, recently, computerized tomography scanning of the brain.

Dr. Benson carries us through these developments most skillfully. An initial presentation of terminology and historical analysis sets the scene for his clear documentation of many classifications. He compares and contrasts his own with these. He indicates how his practical approach is compatible with a useful testing scheme, allowing derivations and conclusions leading to correlations with cerebral pathology. Information related to language development and laterality is clear and succinct. Alexias and agraphias are treated most adequately and gestural-mimetic features are considered. The book also contains most important chapters on psychological effects of aphasia and matters concerned with rehabilitation and its processes. The bibliography is encyclopedic.

New Haven, 1979   Gilbert H. Glaser

CLINICAL NEUROLOGY AND NEUROSURGERY MONOGRAPHS

Volume 1

Editorial Board

Forthcoming Titles in the Series

Fenichel: *Neonatal Neurology*
Glaser: *Temporal Lobe Epilepsy*
Thomas, Stewart and Bundey: *Neurogenetic Disease*
Rudge: *Neuro-otology*
Arnason: *Clinical Neuroimmunology*

Preface

When the editors of this series of neurology monographs first suggested a publication on aphasia, the opportunity seemed excellent. Fifteen years earlier I had arrived at the Boston Veterans Administration Medical Center to study aphasia; preparation of this volume afforded an opportunity to review and record the activities of those years. Dr. Frederick Quadfasel had established an Aphasia Research Center (later called the Neurobehavioral Center) at the BVAMC a few years earlier, and by the time I arrived (1964) four individuals who would achieve distinction in the study of aphasia and related disorders, Norman Geschwind, Harold Goodglass, Edith Kaplan and Robert Sparks, were already in action. Working with them at the Aphasia Research Center provided a constantly stimulating environment with strong emphasis on the observation and evaluation of language-disturbed patients. The tutelage of these four eminent investigators is reflected throughout this volume and, while they cannot be held responsible for any specific statements (quite frankly, each disagrees with certain ideas and interpretations presented in this volume), their work and teachings are gratefully acknowledged. Over the years each of the four has followed a notably different route in their research on aphasia and related disorders and each has continued to influence the Aphasia Research Center.

Soon after arriving at the Aphasia Research Center my task became, and remained, that of a physician responsible for the medical and neurologic disorders underlying the brain disorder that had produced aphasia. Along with this clinical duty, the performance of neuroanatomical localizing studies on the aphasic patients was a continuing project. In other words, the clinical and neurologic aspects of aphasia became my specific responsibility within the group, a division of interest that dictates the dominant theme for this volume. Emphasis has been focused on the clinical aspects of aphasia, on the problems that are pertinent to the practicing neurologist. Because of this it has been impossible to provide adequate coverage of the innumerable fascinating language theories currently and previously popular in the study of aphasia. Specifically, most psychologic, linguistic and anatomic approaches to language function have not been presented. The concentration on the clinical aspects of aphasia presented in this volume is not so much by design, however, as it is a representation of the author's interests and knowledge. Thus, while the influence of each of my four mentors appears throughout this book, only a limited portion of their interests are included, notably those with clinical relevance.

In addition, my experience at the Aphasia Research Center has been influenced and enriched by close association with a series of physicians, called Fellows but more appropriately termed fellow workers. Each Fellow has provided fresh clinical insights based on his personal background and training plus the value of his own considerable abilities to observe. Most have maintained an interest in aphasia and related disorders since leaving the Neurobehavioral Center and many are still in contact with the author. Their efforts are also reflected throughout this volume, and, while the list of Fellows is lengthy, each has influenced the material presented in this book sufficiently to deserve individual recognition. The Fellows of the Neurobehavioral Center include (in alphabetical order): Martin Albert, Michael Alexander, Francois Boller, Jason Brown, Russell Butler, John Carter, Jeffrey Cummings, Martha Denckla, Franco Denis; William Durward, Alvin Fort, Steven Gerson, John Greenberg, Samuel Greenblatt, Paul Hardy, Andrew Kertesz, Theodor Landis, Aubrey Lieberman, Stephen LoVerme, Alan Mandell, Robert Marin, Richard Mayeux, John Meadows, Amos Nahor, David Neary, Tao O, Prather Palmer, David Rosenfield, Eliot Ross, Alan Rubens, Jeffrey Samuels, Benjamin Seltzer, Richard Strub, Bruce Tomlinson, Donald Urrea, Theodore Von Stockert, William Weir and Astushi Yamadori. In addition to the physician-Fellows, a number of nonphysicians with both interest and expertise in aphasia have worked closely with and influenced the Aphasia unit. These include David Howes, Margaret Naeser, David Patton, Marius Mairuszewski, Mel Barton, Howard Gardner, Sheila Blumstein, Frank Spellacy, Barbara Efron, Nancy Helm, Barbara Barresi and Michael Walsh. Over the years a sizable and constantly changing group of medical students, interns, residents and graduate and postgraduate students, research assistants and visiting specialists have spent time at the Aphasia Research Center and many have provided insight and information of value. The intellectual stimulation has been rich; unfortunately, only a portion of it can be recorded in this volume.

Very special acknowledgment must be accorded several individuals whose efforts for this volume are particularly appreciated. Michael Alexander reviewed the entire manuscript in an early stage and provided valuable advice. Without the Herculean efforts of Ms. Ada Jacobs, administrative secretary of the Aphasia Research Center, this book would have been years in the writing. Finally, my wife, Donna, not only produced most of the drawings but, far more important, provided the understanding support necessary for completion of this volume.

Contents

I BACKGROUND

II SYNDROMOLOGY OF APHASIA

III NEUROANATOMICAL CORRELATES OF
SELECTED LANGUAGE FUNCTIONS

IV CLINICAL ASPECTS OF APHASIA

1

Introduction

Aphasia—the loss or impairment of language caused by brain damage.

Alexia—the loss or impairment of the ability to comprehend written or printed language caused by brain damage.

Agraphia—the loss or impairment of the ability to express language in written or printed form caused by brain damage.

With only minor variations in wording, the above definitions are acceptable to (and used by) most individuals dealing with the subject of aphasia. Despite this widespread appearance of agreement, aphasia was born of controversy, has a history of controversy and, to this day, remains a controversial topic. Beyond being the source of lively debate through much of its history, aphasia has also been the source of disagreement, sometimes downright acrimonious. Rather than discussed, viewpoints on aphasia have often been argued. Present day investigators appear increasingly able to accept and many actually utilize divergent points of view, but a tendency remains for viewpoints on aphasia to be argued.

Much of the controversy can be traced directly to the definition of aphasia; not what aphasia is but what it represents. Most aphasiologists agree that aphasia is an impairment of language function and that it occurs following brain damage. The difficulty and the controversy stem from what is meant by the word *language*. This problem must be faced before a meaningful discussion of aphasia can be presented.

APPROACHES TO LANGUAGE AND APHASIA

Language is a widely used term and has accumulated a number of remarkably divergent connotations, many of which are not germane to a discussion of aphasia. Some recognition of the wide variety of approaches to this term used by individuals and groups studying language, however, is crucial to avoid semantic quibbling while concentrating on the consistent features of aphasia. Merely listing some current approaches will highlight the problem, and against this background a working definition of language can be offered for the present volume.

Even excluding the major uses of the word, the study of literature and national tongues, there are many scholarly disciplines with major interest in language and more and more investigators in these disciplines are utilizing

1

aphasia as a research tool. For instance, as aphasia is defined as a problem of language, it has been stated, emphatically and reasonably, that aphasia is the province of the linguist (Jakobson, 1964). Following this line of reasoning several contemporary linguistic subspecialties such as psycholinguistics and neurolinguistics look upon aphasia as a major tool for investigation. In the style of the time, theoretical models of linguistic function are devised and the features of aphasia used to support or refute the model. Increasingly, linguistic attributes highlighted by the study of aphasia are built into the original model of language.

Language is also a mental function, however, and the study of mental functions is the forum of psychology. Any number of psychological subspecialties have developed major interests in communication, verbal symbolism, language development and other language oriented topics and, with increasing frequency, utilize abnormal language (aphasia) for investigative work. Students of developmental psychology have carefully charted the development of language and utilize the loss of language in childhood to derive and support theories of language. Both experimental psychologists and learning theory specialists utilize aphasia to study aspects of their specific spheres and, conversely, offer explanations for the features of language disturbance on the basis of their models. The most directly involved of the psychological subspecialties in the study of aphasia is the comparatively recent subdiscipline known as neuropsychology. Much of the research effort of neuropsychology investigates the residual mental functions of damaged brains; aphasia ranks as one of the most important arenas for neuropsychological investigation. In all psychological approaches, theories of mental function are both the tools and the product; in general, all of the psychological subdisciplines accept the definition of aphasia given above, but the definitions of the word language currently being concocted is vast, materially adding to the confusion surrounding aphasia.

In addition to the direct concern of the linguist and psychologist, many other academic specialists have serious if somewhat more tangential interests in language and aphasia. In the belief that language and thought are intimately intertwined, if not identical, philosophers have long held a strong interest in language and, to a considerably lesser degree, the impairment of language. Philosophical postulations on the relationship of language and thought have been produced for centuries and are still being developed (Popper and Eccles, 1977; Arendt, 1978). Language as an attribute of the mind remains a contemporary theme which affects the composite definition of the word language.

Based on the observation that the brain is of paramount importance to speech and language, neuroscientists such as neuroanatomists, neurophysiologists, neuropathologists, neurochemists and others include language in their investigations of brain function and may utilize pathologically derived language breakdown as a research tool. In fact, almost all anatomical and physiological theories of language function derive directly from observations of aphasia.

In a more practical approach, aphasia produces a disturbance in verbal output, the function usually called speech, and has become a major concern of the academic and clinical subspecialty known as speech pathology. Although they entered the field comparatively late, speech pathologists have demonstrated a remarkable interest in aphasia in recent years. The speech pathologists have propagated their full share of theories of language function, consistent with their highly specialized approach to language through speech. In many institutions speech pathology was spawned from schools of education; this, plus the obvious educational aspects of retraining an aphasic to communicate, has attracted educators into the field, providing a particularly rich source of new theories linking language and human learning.

As aphasia produces an abnormality of human behavior, frequently resulting in serious adjustment problems, many psychiatrists have expressed interest in the subject. Work in this sphere has been somewhat limited in recent years because disturbed language function interferes with the more currently popular psychoanalytically oriented investigations, but younger psychiatrists are developing broader interests including organic mental problems such as aphasia. Psychiatrists have contributed to the study of aphasia for many years and psychiatrically influenced ideas on the meaning of the term *language* are of importance.

Finally, aphasia is a product of brain damage and, as such, falls within the scope of the neurologist. Aphasia was a major factor in the early development of neurology as a medical specialty and remains a crucial link to the understanding of the neurological basis of behavior. Language as an operation of the nervous system is yet another different but acceptable approach to the term.

Each group mentioned above has obvious and legitimate reasons for studying aspects of aphasia based on their interests in either brain or language function. As a result, broad varieties of fascinating approaches to language and aphasia exist and, although very different, each is of significance. Many of the approaches overlap and, altogether too frequently, a theory of language derived from one approach may disagree or be competitive with the theory of another group. Thus, while language is a widely studied subject, considerable disagreement remains over what is meant by the term. Aphasia, as a breakdown of language, is continually drawn into controversy to support or refute theoretical models of language function. Since its inception as a separate topic, aphasia has always occupied a position as pawn in the complex process of the human brain attempting to understand one of its own most important attributes, language. The controversies involve aphasia far less than they do the theories of language function. Nonetheless, as the most promising avenue for approaching the unknown, aphasia has been studied far more intensely as a tool of theorists than as a clinical entity. A purely clinical approach to aphasia is significant for its own sake and, in purest form, is only loosely related to the more academic approaches. Unfortunately, aphasia has proved difficult to discuss without a theory of language function and most clinical reports have also developed or supported some postulate of language organization. The clinical studies have generated their own quota of disagreement.

Against this background the present volume is designed to provide clinical information concerning asphasia for the use of the practicing neurologist. Although the origins of aphasia and many of the subsequent investigations have been the products of neurologists, clinical observations have received comparatively little emphasis. Purely clinical descriptions of aphasia are quite different from scholarly theories of language. This point can be illustrated by a short anecdote. Following a presentation of some basic clinical-neuroanatomical correlations of aphasia, a young psychologist in the audience stated that while fascinated by the topic he could not agree with the theory presented. In the view of the neurologist giving the presentation no theory had been presented. Rather, the talk had been limited to observations from the speaker's clinical experience abetted by material gleaned from a century-long reservoir of pertinent medical reports. If the theories held by the psychologist did not agree with the clinical data, these theories needed serious reevaluation as they were inconsistent with actual observations.

The anecdote highlights one major intention of this volume. Theoretical model-building, in this instance a model of language, is an accepted technique of scientific investigation, almost essential for the "soft" sciences. In this technique, a theory or model of a given function is postulated and then tested against observations that are usually derived from specifically fashioned experimental tests. Observations in support of a theory are welcomed and even proof that a theory is incorrect represents a scientific gain by adding additional hard knowledge toward understanding a function. The model-building approach is far removed from the approach of clinical medicine, however. The clinician evaluates his patient by correlating data about physical malfunction with observations provided by physical examination and laboratory testing, all combined to make a diagnosis (theory). While the clinician's findings may be helpful to the scientific model builders as a source of data, the clinical observations are far more important as guides for the clinical management of the patient.

This book is designed to present as much useful clinical-observation information as possible and unabashedly utilizes a localizationist approach to aphasia. The information presented here is not offered to confirm or refute any present or past theory of language. Rather it represents a compendium of clinical observations from the author's experience and from the world literature, excluding, as completely as practicable, theories of language function. Most neurological literature on aphasia has been presented in terms which support one or another theory of language function. Taken individually most such presentations are understandable; in total, however, the aphasia literature presents so many conflicting theories that coherence is sacrificed. The aphasia literature is notorious for the confusion of its terminology and its theories. Insofar as possible, theoretical aspects will be omitted from this volume and clinical observations will be emphasized. Aphasia, however, is of multidisciplinary interest and valuable information concerning language function comes from many sources. Some of this nonclinical data, considered valuable for the practicing clinician, will be included.

The present volume, therefore, has two purposes. The basic goal is to aid practicing clinicians in caring for patients with aphasia. As a secondary function, it can be anticipated that some of the information offered will prove useful for scientists investigating language. It must be recognized that the body of information reported here is woefully incomplete; much additional information is constantly being added and this enlarging corpus should allow for both improved theories of language and better care for the aphasic patient.

DEFINITIONS

Based on the varied approaches to aphasia it can be expected that individual investigators would define the bàsic terms idiosyncratically, producing subtle but significant differences. This is generally true, and to counteract this problem most terms will be defined as they appear, using context as an aid to understanding the meaning. Several primary terms, however, demand definition at the outset.

Aphasia

As already noted, there is comparatively little disagreement over the definition of aphasia itself. Many different authors (Nielsen, 1936; Benson and Geschwind, 1971; Darley, 1975; Adams and Victor, 1977) present almost identical definitions that can be paraphrased as: *aphasia is the loss or impairment of language caused by brain damage.* More detailed definitions can also be made. For instance, Darley, Aronson and Brown (1975) described aphasia as "a multimodality reduction in the capacity to decode (interpret) and encode (formulate) meaningful linguistic elements . . . It is manifested in difficulties in listening, reading, speaking and writing." The basic meaning remains similar, however, and, as already noted, the controversy centers on the meaning of language, not the meaning of aphasia.

Language, Speech and Thought

These three terms have been given many definitions, most differing only slightly, based on the interests of the individuals offering the definition. Most such definitions prove useful for one group but have limited relevance for others and often prove confusing to the clinician. In an attempt to obviate this problem operational definitions will be introduced for these three key activities. Specifically, an attempt will be made to separate, functionally, speech, language and thought. Without separation (and most contemporary investigators carefully avoid making such a separation) the resulting overlap proves discouragingly confusing.

Speech can be described as the mechanical portion of an individual's ability to communicate with oral language, demanding the combination of the appropriate neuromuscular actions necessary for phonation and articulation. Pure speech disorders, often called dysarthria, are disturbances of this neuromuscular apparatus producing abnormalities of articulation and phonation. Some authorities include the abilities to write and gesture when discussing speech, but for present purposes speech will be limited to the activities of oral communication. Clinically, there are many examples of speech disturbance with absolutely no disturbance of either language or thought. An obvious example is the severe bulbar paralysis in cases of poliomyelitis or amyotrophic lateral sclerosis causing severe hypophonia or even mutism. While the loss of speech is extreme, there is no true problem with language. If a substitute means of communication can be established, the patient will respond adequately, demonstrating appropriate language function. Another common example is the rigidity seen in advanced parkinsonism which may interfere with the mechanics of verbal output so seriously that no output occurs, but again no language problem need be present. Many other examples of pure speech loss are commonly recognized in the clinic. From an operational view then, speech can be pathologically involved without either language or thought disturbance being present.

While *language* can be separated from the purely mechanical act of speech rather easily, a simple description of language proves difficult. Some consider language the ability to communicate through the use of symbols. A disturbance of language would incorporate disturbance in the ability to comprehend (decode) and/or program (encode) the symbols necessary for communication. Aphasia is the classic clinical example of a language disturbance and, while frequently combined with either speech or thought disorder, aphasia can occur as a pure language abnormality.

Thought, the third entity, is the most resistant of all to description. A number of philosophers insist that language and thought cannot be separated (Merleau-Ponty, 1964; Arendt, 1978). In clinical experience, however, a number of features imply a distinction between language and thought, at least on an operational level. Just as relatively pure speech or language disorders can be seen clinically, certain disease states represent relatively pure "thought disorders," for instance, schizophrenia in many of its forms produces a characteristically abnormal verbal output in which there is neither speech nor language defect. Thus the paranoid schizophrenic may manifest unbelievably bizarre patterns of thought, but express them with excellent speech and full language competency. Similarly, severely depressed patients show seriously disordered thinking but little or no problem expressing their morbid thoughts. In some stages of dementia significant deficiencies in thinking can be demonstrated in patients whose language output is relatively competent; in later stages, however, many dements also show significant language problems. It is not unusual for a patient with early Alzheimer changes to have an adequate vocabulary and normal syntactic structures while showing seriously deficient cognitive abilities.

Disturbances of communication via writing (agraphia) and gesture (body language) are common in clinical practice. Just as with vocalized verbal output, the disturbance in these two spheres may be based on peripheral motor (speech) problems (e.g. pseudobulbar palsy) or central ideational (thought) disturbance (e.g. catatonia) but pure language disturbance can and often does underlie abnormalities of writing and gesture.

In clinical practice some mixture of symptoms relating to speech, language and thought is almost constant. The pure states are comparatively rare. Thus, most patients with aphasic disorders have problems in two or even all three categories. Nonetheless, clinical experience demonstrates that speech, language and thought can be affected separately and it would appear that each has separate significance. Both clinicians and clinical investigators should keep this separation clearly in mind. By definition, and for clarity of thinking, aphasia is a disturbance of language, not a disturbance of thinking capability or speech (Benson, 1975). In the frequent situation in which a language disturbance is coupled with either speech or thought disturbance, the combination should be carefully noted as both prognosis and therapy techniques depend on the combination of problems.

Other terms will be discussed in the context of the clinical syndromes, but before detailing the syndromes some general background information deserves review.

LATERALIZATION OF LANGUAGE FUNCTION

One of the more dramatic findings in aphasia (and all of biology for that matter) concerns the well-known fact that in the majority of humans a single cerebral hemisphere, the left, almost totally controls the major function of language. This unique characteristic is of such enormous significance in the discussion of localized language functions that it warrants presentation as a separate chapter (see Ch. 14). Left hemisphere dominance for language is a basic fact that must be accepted and remembered: *for almost every right-handed and for many left-handed adults, the left hemisphere subserves all or most of the functions of language.*

CHILDHOOD LANGUAGE ABNORMALITY

Abnormalities of language in childhood and the term *childhood aphasia* have been confusing and controversial for many years. Without question, language abnormality occurs frequently in childhood but the clinical picture of childhood language abnormality often fails to fit the descriptions of aphasia presented here and, quite realistically, represents a totally different clinical problem. Two major divisions of childhood language abnormality should be recognized, one a *developmental language problem* and the second an *acquired aphasia of childhood*. This division highlights the total difference in the basic problems. Children with developmental language problems have never developed normal language and, therefore, fall outside the accepted definition of aphasia as they have never had language to be lost or impaired. Inasmuch as their language symptoms are based on developmental abnormality rather than focal cerebral damage, neither the clinical features nor the anatomical correlations are necessarily the same as those of acquired aphasia. It would be preferable for this disorder to be called *language retardation* with the term *childhood aphasia* reserved for children who have developed language in a normal fashion but, following brain damage, show language abnormality.

Children who have begun to develop language can sustain a language disturbance following a cerebral insult and the result is, at least in general appearance, analogous to the acquired aphasias of adults (Guttman, 1942). There are several characteristic differences of the acquired aphasia of childhood, however. First, cerebral dominance for language apparently develops with advancing age. The younger the child at the onset of acquired aphasia, the less complete the dominance for language in one hemisphere and the better the other hemisphere can assume language function. Zangwill (1960) called this an "equipotentiality" of the two hemispheres for language in young children. Many investigators believe that some ability for the other hemisphere to assume language is retained through the first ten or twelve years of life and possibly well beyond (Smith, 1966; Lenneberg, 1967; Cummings and Benson, 1979).

A second distinctive characteristic is that the younger the child at the time of onset the more rapid and more complete the recovery from acquired aphasia. Careful testing suggests that language function is never quite as full in a child who recovers aphasia secondary to a damaged dominant hemisphere (Lenneberg, 1967; Hecaen, 1976) although it is often sufficient for normal use. With increasing age, the time necessary to recover language function increases; a child aged three or four with an acquired aphasia may speak within a few weeks or a month while the child of ten or twelve may wait many months before return of significant language function. Obviously, both the rate and the degree of recovery reflect the severity of cerebral damage and, of course, the presence of bilateral damage compounds the problem. The ability of the nondominant hemisphere to assume some or much language function continues for some time after onset of aphasia and may continue well beyond the age of five years (Krashen, 1973) to twelve years (Lenneberg, 1967) usually suggested. Many young men who became aphasic following brain injury sustained in combat made excellent language recovery. In general, aphasics aged twenty to thirty years have a better prognosis than those fifty or sixty years old. Before simply accepting advancing age as the key feature, however, attention must be given to the cause of the aphasia. Trauma, which in general has a better prognosis, is the more common cause of aphasia in the young while vascular and neoplastic problems with graver outlook predominate in later years (see Ch. 3). It still appears, however, that the lower the age of onset of aphasia, the faster and more complete the improvement and this is most notably seen in the young, developing child.

A third significant difference of childhood aphasia concerns the fluency of verbal output (see Ch. 4). It is often stated that the child who acquires aphasia never shows a fluent, paraphasic, jargon type of verbal output. This may not be true in the absolute, but the vast majority of children with acquired aphasia produce a nonfluent verbal output. Most children with acquired aphasia are initially mute (a relatively rare happening in the adult) and in the initial recovery stages the verbal output is characteristically slow, sparse and hypophonic. Nonfluent language output appears characteristic for all acquired aphasias of childhood, regardless of the site of brain insult.

Finally, one additional but exceedingly troublesome problem in the evaluation of acquired aphasia in childhood concerns the stages of language development. The quantity and complexity of language available to the child increase with increasing age, a crucial factor in the evaluation of language loss in the child. There is, however, a tremendous variation in language ability among individual children of any given age, based on intelligence, language use in the home, language used by siblings or friends, educational experiences and recognized variations in cerebral development. Sufficient brain damage to produce an acquired aphasia not only damages acquired language capabilities unevenly but also delays normal language development. Coupled with the tremendous variability of verbal competency of childhood these additional factors pose enormous difficulties for the clinician attempting to correlate the language of an aphasic child with a normal "expectation." The standard procedure is to compare the aphasic child's language with normal adult function, note the deficits but disregard those language functions usually unavailable to a child of that age. At best this produces a crude guess. Clear demonstration of the amount of language lost by a child is extremely difficult.

The pathology underlying childhood language problems deserves separate mention. A variety of developmental abnormalities of the cerebral hemispheres can produce language retardation. Some are actual structural changes, most often involving the temporal and/or parietal lobes. Based on the equipotentiality of the hemispheres for language, it can be conjectured that bilateral cerebral pathology underlies language retardation. One important factor is that a child cannot learn to use language if language cannot be comprehended. Deafness provides an important source of developmental language problems. If the deafness is peripheral, corrective measures can be instituted and are the primary task of deaf training. If, however, the deafness is based on a central abnormality, the child will respond poorly, if at all, to standard deaf-training techniques and a serious language retardation will be present. One of the few carefully studied cases of developmental language retardation to come to postmortem study (Landau, Goldstein, and Kleffner, 1960) had developmental abnormality of the central auditory system causing a "central deafness" and a severe language retardation, intractable to available training techniques.

In contrast, the acquired aphasia of childhood stems from many different pathological sources, generally analogous to the causes of aphasia in adults (see Ch. 3). The most common etiology of acquired childhood aphasia is trauma but other sources such as infection, tumor and even cerebral vascular accident are seen regularly. Prior to the widespread use of antibiotics, cerebral abscess in the temporal lobe complicating a chronic otitis media was a common cause of aphasia. Acquired aphasia is not common in childhood but certainly does occur and, in general, shows characteristics similar to the aphasias of adult life that will be described in detail.

The prognosis for developmental language disturbance must remain guarded at present. Techniques are being developed that attempt treatment of inborn language disturbance with some claim to success but the problem remains severe. Fortunately, with advancing age and maturation of the nervous system, many children with language retardation develop compensatory mechanisms which allow some degree of communication. The prognosis in acquired aphasia is considerably better. As already noted, the younger the child, the more likely that the other hemisphere can assume the function of language. Unfortunately, bilateral hemispheric damage is not uncommon and seriously impairs the recovery potential. Thus, in individual cases, prognosis must be guarded, at least until the course reveals evidence of recovery. Fortunately, most children who acquire aphasia do regain a useful degree of language function and many recover a surprising ability to use language competently.

APHASIA IN POLYGLOTS

Individuals who are fluent in several languages present an interesting problem when they become aphasic. Which of the multiple languages will recover? A tendency for one language to recover better than the others has been recorded with sufficient frequency to warrant discussion (Paradis, 1972). Some polyglot aphasics become functional in one language but remain totally aphasic in their other language(s). Ribot's Rule (1883) posits that the language best recovered by the polyglot should be the mother tongue. This is based on the observation that with memory disturbance (amnesia) information learned early in life is retrieved better than more recently acquired information. Another early postulation concerning the recovery of language by polyglots, often called Pitres' Law (1895), states that the language that the patient used most before onset of aphasia will be recovered best, even if it is not the first learned. Neither rule has been validated, and, in fact, both are "honored as much by being broken as by being followed" (Hecaen and Albert, 1978).

In an excellent discussion of the recovery of language function by the polyglot, Goldstein (1948) emphasized three factors: 1) Some polyglots are truly fluent only in one (usually the mother) tongue and recovery of other previously known languages tends to be limited. There are exceptions to this observation (Hinshelwood, 1900) but it applies to a majority of polyglot aphasics. 2) More than one language may recover but the recovery level may be uneven. Goldstein states that "the patient will try to use that language which appears best for his purpose," possibly to the exclusion of the others. Careful testing of truly polyglot aphasics in their several languages, however, usually reveals at least some degree of function in each. Similarly, the characteristics of aphasia demonstrated in one language are usually demonstrable in the other(s). 3) Dialect seriously confuses the picture of recovery by a polyglot aphasic. As dialect is more often dependent upon the motor or phonetic qualities of verbal output it may be differentially lost or retained in aphasia, complicating but not reflecting the underlying loss or retention of language. Goldstein concludes that multiple factors determine the pattern of language recovery of an aphasic polyglot and, in general, recovery will reflect the patient's attempt to achieve the best communication system available.

Observation suggests that one important factor in determining the first language to be recovered by a polyglot is the language milieu available during recovery. In French-Canada many citizens are bilingual but most hospitals emphasize one of the two languages; the language recovered by aphasics in these circumstances is often the language used in the specific hospital (Lambert, Fillebaum, 1959). This also varies with the factors posited by Goldstein (patients who primarily knew and used only one language generally recovered this one best) and by whether the two languages were learned and used in a single environment (compound languages) or in separate environments (coordinate languages). The latter were more often dissociated during recovery.

Some observers posit that variations in the recovery of separate languages by a polyglot are based on lesion localization, a premise which has been emphatically denied for many years (Pitres, 1895; Goldstein, 1948). Occasional cases supporting at least some anatomically based differences continue to surface, however (Bychowski, 1919; Obler and Albert, 1977). The most dramatic examples involve written language, particularly when the two languages utilize strikingly different methods of writing (Indo-European, Chinese, Arabic) (Sasanuma and Fujimura, 1971; Yamadori, 1975; Obler and Albert, 1977). That lesion location may be a factor in differential recovery is not totally unacceptable but is only one of multiple factors and, in our present state of knowledge, does not appear to be the factor of greatest importance (Albert and Obler, 1978).

Aphasia in polylinguals offers, in a microcosm, a glimpse of the multiplicity of factors influencing the overall picture of aphasia. Just as the simplicities of Ribot's and Pitres' Rules were insufficient to characterize polyglot aphasia, so the many models of language function, past and present (and for the foreseeable future), fail to explain adequately the clinical findings in aphasia. Insofar as possible this volume will be restricted to descriptions and observations of aphasia plus discussion of some of the many extraneous factors influencing aphasia. Readers desiring theories of language function to "explain" the symptoms of aphasia can seek satisfaction in almost every paper, monograph and book ever produced on the subject. In fact, most individual papers on the subject emphasize theoretically devised interpretations of language function. The present volume will feature a more confined picture, omitting theories in favor of clinical observations.

2

Historical Background

Formal delineation and study of aphasia is only a bit over a century old, but the material produced has been massive in quantity, fascinating and significant. As already noted, much early work either developed or was dependent upon theories of language function. Most of the major figures in the history of aphasia produced and are best known for attempted explanations of communication through language. This is well recorded in many excellent resumés of the history of aphasia, almost without exception slanted in the direction of the author's theoretical bias. Taken as a group, however, the reviews provide a tremendous quantity of excellently abstracted background information. In the following section only selected portions of this vast array can be presented, and without doubt the material chosen reflects the author's interests. For additional historical background and particularly for outlines of the many diverse theoretical explanations of language function the reader is referred to a number of excellent papers and chapters. Particularly recommended are the historical resumés of Freud (1891), Head (1926), Weisenburg and McBride (1933), Benton and Joynt (1960), Brain (1961), Geschwind (1967 c), Quadfasel (1968), Cole (1968) and Hecaen and Albert (1978).

The extensive historical survey by Benton and Joynt (1960) of pre-Broca efforts in aphasia clearly demonstrates that a wide variety of language disorders had been noted for many centuries prior to the major thrust of aphasia study. In fact, Benton and Joynt aver that most of the commonly accepted language disorders were well described prior to 1860. Nonetheless, the study of aphasia, as presently recognized, dates from 1861.

The relationship between the mind (mental activities) and the brain had evolved and been debated over the centuries. By the early 19th century two clearly dissimilar beliefs about the brain's function in language production had crystalized. Some investigators, taking their lead from the early phrenologists such as Gall and Spurzheim maintained that specific mental functions were subserved by specific areas of the brain. This viewpoint was carried to the extreme of denoting various mental functions (love, pride, greed, speech, etc.) and suggesting specific areas of the brain as centers for these behaviors. Staunch opponents to this extreme "localization" viewpoint believed that mental function was a product of the entire brain working as a unit and that mental ability was a reflection of total brain volume. They were unwilling to accept the suggestion that specific areas of the brain were responsible for performing specific mental activities.

As a part of this long-standing debate, a primitive skull was demonstrated to an anthropological meeting in Paris early in 1861 with an implication of a direct relationship between the surmised mental limitations of the subject and the distinctly small brain volume. A lively controversy developed as to whether a direct relationship existed between brain size and brain function. At this time a patient of one physician-member of the society became "speechless" and then died. Postmortem studies revealed a large frontal lesion and the physician, Paul Broca, submitted this case as evidence favoring the localization viewpoint (1861). Broca suggested that, inasmuch as the patient had become speechless following frontal brain damage, "speech" could be localized in the posterior-inferior portion of the frontal lobe, at least in this single case. Obviously, this direct statement produced further disagreement but also encouraged reporting of additional cases of speechlessness (aphasia). Some of the studied cases supported, others failed to support, Broca's localization.

The inclusion of clinical case material in what had previously been an exclusively academic debate greatly stimulated interest in the pathology underlying impaired language. From this surge of interest stem, both directly and indirectly, most past and many present currents in the study of aphasia. In addition, the interest in aphasia coincided with and strongly influenced the development of clinical neurology as a medical specialty. From the localizationist-influenced subspecialty of neurology, two other subspecialties, psychiatry and neurosurgery, inherited much of their original direction (both Freud and Foerster were well-trained neurologists before they became creative pioneers in the fields of psychiatry and neurosurgery respectively). Thus, a single case presented to a scholarly discussion group exerted an influence far beyond the value of the case.

Several years after presenting his original material, Broca called the attention of the medical world to the fact that only the left hemisphere appeared to be involved when language was impaired (1865). He reported that the brains of patients who had become "speechless" had cerebral pathology located in the left hemisphere whereas patients with pathology involving the same areas of the right hemisphere did not become "speechless." It is now generally accepted that this dramatic finding had been reported some twenty-five years earlier by Dax (1836) but his paper was not published and his report remained virtually unknown until Broca's observations had been published. Chapter 14 contains additional details concerning the hemispheric lateralization of language function in the human brain. From the date of Broca's original report, the study of aphasia and its correlation with neuroanatomical localization has continued and remains the focus of considerable disagreement.

The second major advance in the localizationist approach to aphasia followed publication of the doctoral thesis of a young German medical student, Karl Wernicke, in 1874. Wernicke posited two distinct types of aphasia, motor and sensory, which were clinically separable and supported his theory with clinical-pathological correlation. Wernicke later postulated a third variety of aphasia (which he called *conduction aphasia*), based upon a diagrammatic outline of portions of the brain participating in language function. Following

Wernicke's initial presentation, both the clinical-pathological localization of the varieties of aphasia and the use of diagrams to "explain" language disturbances in aphasia became increasingly popular. Within a few years a plethora of schemes and classifications of aphasia appeared (Lichtheim, 1885; Charcot, 1877; Bastian, 1898). Most subsequent work purporting localization of language functions in designated areas of the brain has utilized the format devised by the 19th-century continental neurologists who followed Wernicke's original postulation. The localizationists claimed that specific areas of the brain (centers) were essential for specific language functions as "proved" by the correlation of specific language disturbances during life with postmortem demonstration of pathology located at specific sites. The clinical findings of aphasia were usually expressed in the psychophilosophical jargon of the day (auditory images, sentence schemes, verbal amnesia, mind blindness, etc.) and the clinical-anatomical localizations usually referred to the effect of focal cerebral pathology on these hypothesized functions. Thus a glossokinetic center, a writing center, an auditory verbal image center and many similar concoctions were postulated and "demonstrated" by clinical-pathological correlations. Among the many contributors to this early approach to aphasia several deserve note because of their influence: these include Lichtheim (1885), Charcot (1889), Bastian (1898), Kleist (1934) and Nielson (1936). Of special note in the clinical-anatomical localization approach was the work of Henschen (1922) who collected every published case of aphasia in the literature (1,337) with sufficient information to allow a clinical-pathological correlation. Henschen's is a truly monumental work but was published too late to exert any significant influence or gain the respect deserved.

Most of the localizationists worked in the latter part of the 19th century and the early part of the 20th century, a period which saw the development and flowering of the clinical-pathological approach in all aspects of medicine. This approach influenced medical science tremendously but, without question, had limitations. The limitations in the language disturbances became increasingly apparent as the number of classificatory schemes increased. Excesses in the claims of the localizationists (in particular, basing major theories on a single case) became, and remain, obvious, just as many of the functions that were correlated with pathology would not presently be accepted as language functions. The localizationist viewpoint deserved and received considerable criticism and eventually lost credibility.

During the period of the clinical-pathological correlations, a sizable group of scholars steadfastly adhered to another, quite different, view of language disturbances, advocating a more holistic, universal approach. One of the earliest and eventually one of the most influential proponents was John Hughlings Jackson (1864), the English neurologist who considered aphasia from a dynamic, psychological viewpoint rather than as a static, neuroanatomical correlation. Jackson's opinions were neither understood nor accepted for many years but eventually attained considerable influence. Sigmund Freud, in a monograph on aphasia published in 1891, was strongly influenced by Jackson and roundly criticized the "diagram makers." His monograph received scant attention (it sold only 257 copies in ten years) and it was not until the dramatic presentations of Pierre Marie in 1906 that the holistic point of view influenced a wide audience. Marie presented a paper provocatively entitled "The Third Frontal Convolution Does Not Play any Special Role in the Function of Language," which reopened the old disagreement. Another debate, not dissimilar to the 1861 discussions, took place in Paris with Dejerine, a proponent of the classical localizationist view, opposing Marie's broader, more holistic viewpoint. While the result was, typically, unresolved, the influence of the holistic approach on aphasia steadily increased from that point and numbered many significant advocates over the early part of the 20th century. They included Head (1926), Kinnear Wilson (1926), Pick (1931), Isserlin (1929, 1931, 1932) and more recently Weisenburg and McBride (1935), Wepman (1951), Bay (1964), Schuell (1964) and Critchley (1970).

Henry Head (1926) outlined a clinical-psychological approach to aphasia and included himself as an example of those using this approach. Many aphasiologists, both past and present, whose efforts can be accurately described as clinical-psychological, recognize that pathological damage to certain neuroanatomical locations is consistently associated with certain types of aphasic symptomatology but their approach to language emphasizes psychologic and linguistic evidence rather than neurologic or anatomic findings. Most of the "holists" mentioned in the previous paragraph utilized a psychological correlation approach to the clinical problems of aphasia.

In a somewhat different manner, some aphasiologists have retained a total unwillingness to accept specific localization for aphasia syndromes. One notable example is Von Monakow (1914, 1928) who has stated that there is no aphasia, but only aphasic patients. He postulated that all cerebral pathology is accompanied by a large and variable surrounding area of malfunction (diaschisis), the source of the variable clinical patterns of aphasia. He accepted that damage to the language areas of the brain was the source of true aphasia but recognized only motor and sensory variations and considered that diaschisis could involve such variable portions of the brain as to make localization of language malfunction in a given individual impossible. In a similar way, the gestalt psychologists, best exemplified by Goldstein (1948) and Conrad (1954), promoted a holistic approach to language loss. Brain damage interfered with the basic function of language (gestalten), with the variable aphasic symptomatology derived from variations in the disturbances of total cerebral organization. The gestalt approach substituted psychological concepts for neuroanatomically based theories and attained considerable influence in all spheres of psychology including the psychological explanation of language disturbance. Scientific support for the holistic approach also came from the animal experimentation of Lashley (1926). His early work suggested that cerebral function was not the product of a specific neuroanatomical structure but resulted from the integrated participation of large masses of cerebral tissues. Lashley and his followers introduced rigid measuring and observational techniques to psychology, but in the end these studies reaffirmed the importance of specific cerebral structures in psychological functions (1929). While most contemporary students of aphasia cannot accept the fully holistic view of language proposed earlier, some proponents maintain a totally holistic viewpoint and many others accept portions of the dynamic, holistic approach. The influence of these workers remains strong.

While the above discussion suggests two sharply antagonistic approaches to aphasia each with strong proponents, almost every student of aphasia has held views and made observations supportive of both approaches; only the overview is different. Identical case material has been described by aphasiologists of the two schools, leading to strikingly diverse postulations of language defect which, on careful evaluation, are not incompatible. Indeed, any number of influential apasiologists are linked with one theoretical approach but have produced meaningful work in the other. For instance, Kurt Goldstein (1948) is recognized as a staunch proponent of the holistic (organismic) approach to aphasia but his works include some of the clearest and best case descriptions available in contemporary literature, often including excellent descriptions of the neuropathology. Similarly, the Russian psychologists headed by Luria (1970) express strong antilocalizationist views but their work features careful descriptions of aphasic syndromes, often correlated with an anatomical localization of pathology. Thus, while it is accurate to divide prevailing approaches to aphasia into the anatomically based localizers and the psychologically based holists, most investigators utilize material from both approaches to a greater or lesser degree.

Interest in aphasia waned considerably in the years preceding and immediately following World War II. Care for the brain-injured aphasia cases of World War II, however, led directly to the introduction of formal aphasia therapy (see Ch. 18) and produced a new specialty, speech pathology, with a major interest in aphasia. In turn, interest in language malfunction by neurologists, psychologists and more recently, linguists, has increased greatly. Some of the older localizationist ideas have been revived and a better integration of neurologic and psychologic approaches to aphasia has resulted. The work of Geschwind (1965) emphasizing cortical-cortical disconnection as a major source of language disorder greatly increased the breadth of the anatomical correlation approach. The works of contemporary Italians, DeRenzi and Vignolo (1962), the French investigators Hecaen (1965) and Lhermitte (1969), the Russians headed by Luria (1966), the Germans Leichsner (1957), Bay (1964) and Poeck (1972) and Americans Goodglass (1972) and Benton (1964) have combined both psychological and anatomical studies. Research in aphasia has burgeoned in the last two decades and while the opposing theoretical viewpoints initiated by the Paris debates of 1861 and heightened by the debates of Marie and Dejerine a half century later remain, there appears to be an increasing ability to bridge the two views.

Finally, in his book *Aphasia and Kindred Disorders,* Henry Head (1926) described the intellectual background of aphasia as "chaos." To this he added his own unique theoretical approach which compounded the chaos. In addition, however, Head also introduced a new tool for the investigation of aphasia, a formal, reproducible series of tests. Weisenburg and McBride (1935), in attempting to replicate Head's work, fashioned a far more complete battery of language function tests and fostered a technique which has developed into a major factor in the understanding of aphasia. Most serious investigations of aphasia (for either clinical or research purposes) now include testing by one or more of the standardized aphasia batteries (see Ch. 4). In most research units, one or many experimental tests are routinely included. Contemporary aphasia research often centers on a test, and explanations of language and language defect are derived from the test results. Not infrequently, the experimental data are inconsistent with clinical observation, a further source of confusion and disagreement. In fact, the evaluation of aphasia has become an important independent aspect of the history of aphasia. The introduction of experimental design has greatly broadened and strengthened the investigation of language function as seen in aphasia and ranks as a major advance.

As a history, this short chapter has been woefully inadequate. Many (in fact, most) individuals of importance in the history of aphasia have not received mention in these pages. Even more conspicuously, the many investigators under whom aphasia research has expanded so explosively in the past decade receive no mention at all, although many will be referenced in the text. It is hoped that this cursory outline will aid the uninitiated in coping with the many confusions and disagreements abounding in the older literature, controversies which still affect contemporary studies.

3

Neuropathological Substrate of Aphasia

By definition aphasia is the product of damage to the brain. By necessity then, a neuropathology of aphasia exists and the type of pathological involvement assumes considerable importance to the neurologist caring for an individual aphasic. The literature on aphasia, particularly in this century, contains surprisingly little specific detail about the pathology, and even reports on the neuroanatomical loci of lesions underlying language loss are more the exception than the rule. There is an obvious place in any study of aphasia for information on the neuropathological substrate underlying the disorder.

As a start, a number of generalizations (observations) can be offered about the pathology of aphasia. First, as clearly stated in the definition, *aphasia is the product of damage to the brain*. This excludes neuropathological processes involving nonbrain portions of the CNS, non-neurological states such as psychologic disorders and, as they do not reflect damage, congenital or developmental abnormalities. Secondly, aphasia can and does occur with any type of neuropathology capable of producing structural alterations in an appropriate portion of the language area, whether this be the cortex, the cortical-cortical connections or the subcortical areas. *It is the neuroanatomic location of the brain damage, not the causative agent, that is the key to the aphasic symptomatology.*

Aphasia may occur with functional CNS disorders such as epilepsy, toxic or metabolic confusional states, dementia, etc. In these conditions the language disorder almost invariably appears with and is usually overshadowed by other serious neurological and behavioral abnormalities. *Whenever aphasia is the outstanding finding of a neurological examination, focal structural pathology involving language area structures should be suspected.*

In company with many other behavioral abnormalities of the CNS, aphasia is not the product of a specific pathology. *Totally different pathological states can and do produce identical aphasic syndromes.* There are certain patterns of residual aphasia symptomatology, however, particularly in the vascular disorders, which suggest specific types of pathology. Thus, the symptom complex of aphasia may be used as a clue by the neurologist searching for the variety of pathology present.

There is *no* aphasia produced by pathology involving organs other than the brain (even the language loss noted in severe confusional states or generalized metabolic toxic disorders involves language by disrupting brain function). There is *almost* no aphasia from nonlanguage area brain involvement. When pathology involves nonlanguage areas of the brain, the aphasic symptoms will either be absent or negligible in comparison to other neurologic findings. This is particularly true of pathology involving the nondominant hemisphere.

For the neurologist, the type of pathology underlying an individual case of aphasia is of obvious significance as he must treat the disease process as well as the aphasia and both the treatment modality chosen and the prognosis will ultimately depend upon the cause of the aphasia. A short review of the varieties of pathology capable of producing aphasia is worthwhile.

VASCULAR DISEASE

A variety of disorders affecting cerebral (or extracranial) blood vessels and secondarily producing damage to selected areas of the brain are among the most common sources of structural alteration suffered by the CNS (Romanul, 1970). Vascular disease is probably the most common single cause of aphasia. Traditionally, three major varieties of vascular pathology, embolism, thrombosis and hemorrhage, are recognized. This traditional breakdown may not be accurately descriptive of all vascular conditions underlying aphasia, but it will be followed for ease of presentation.

Modes of diagnosis of these three disorders have changed with time, producing shifts in suspected incidence and importance. For many years cerebral hemorrhage was the diagnosis given to almost all stroke cases. With more widespread availability of neuropathological studies (autopsies which included examination of the brain) there was as shift towards thrombosis as the most common diagnosis in CVA (Wechsler, 1952). In recent years, particularly following the surgeons' increased ability to perform great vessel surgery, the diagnosis of embolism has increased in popularity, if not in frequency. Currently, the widespread use of computerized tomography as a diagnostic tool has demonstrated that the incidence of small, deep hemorrhages in cases presenting with aphasia is considerably higher than previously suspected.

Whether vascular pathology provides good material for research studies of aphasia has long been a topic of disagreement. Many investigators, particularly those who work in neurosurgical centers where trauma and tumor material predominate, suggest that a stroke rarely involves an otherwise normal brain. They claim that in most instances where vascular disease has caused aphasia there will be evidence of widespread vascular insufficiency and/or multiple infarcts; significant pathology, therefore, will exist outside the site of the vascular accident. Other equally sincere investigators dispute this statement and note that in many cases carefully studied at postmortem, the CNS pathology was limited to the area of the brain served by the involved vessel producing a sharply exact focal lesion. As usual, there is truth on both sides of the controversy; some vascular cases are indeed messy, with multiple areas of damage producing a confusing clinical picture while others appear to have single, precise lesions. For the clinician this argument is of little consequence for there is no disagreement about the fact that vascular pathology is the most common source of aphasia in peacetime medical practice. Whether vascular cases are or are not superior as material for aphasia research, cerebral vascular disease with aphasia as a complicating residual problem is a common problem in the practice of neurology.

Thrombosis

The occlusion of a vessel by alterations in the vessel wall (thrombosis) was once considered the most common cause of acute cerebral vascular disease, and conversely, a stroke was automatic evidence of arteriosclerotic pathology (Wechsler, 1952). Thrombosis is now thought to be less frequent in occurrence and many disease processes other than arteriosclerosis are known to produce thrombosis. In addition to the well-recognized alterations in vessel walls produced by arteriosclerosis and subintimal hemorrhage, inflammatory disorders such as giant cell arteritis, syphilitic endarteritis, polyarteritis nodosa and lupus erythematosis can occlude vessels. Other disorders such as polycythemia, leukemia and sickle cell anemia can alter blood constituents causing cell aggregation and can lead to vessel occlusion. Alterations of cerebral circulation secondary to heart failure, myocardial infarction, cardiac arrythmic, surgical shock, postural hypotension, dehydration and even sleep may lead to occlusion of a compromised vessel. Trauma to one of the great vessels, particularly one of the carotid arteries, can damage the intima and lead to occlusion through either subcortical hemorrhage or as a nidus for cell aggregations. If the vascular territory affected by any of these causes of occlusion involves a significant portion of the language area, aphasia will result.

Embolism

Occlusion of a vessel by material floating in the arterial system was once considered almost exclusively a disease of the young. With widespread use of carotid angiography, retinal vessel visualization and increased understanding of blood coagulation, embolism is now recognized as a frequent and important source of stroke. The potential sources of emboli are remarkably widespread. For years it was believed that almost all emboli came from the heart, small bits of mural thrombosis dislodged from the cardiac wall by auricular fibrillation or other cardiac arrhythmia. Angiography has demonstrated that calcific placques, particularly in the carotid vessels, are frequent sources of cerebral emboli (see Fig. 3-1). Cardiac surgery and bacterial endocarditis are much less common but very real sources of emboli. Occasionally emboli emanate from the lungs or even the great veins, and on rare occasions emboli of tumor cells may become lodged in the vessels of the brain. It has long been recognized that trauma to the long bones can lead to fat emboli which can enter and then occlude cerebral vessels. While the latter conditions are comparatively rare, embolism is now accepted as a frequent type of aphasia-producing pathology.

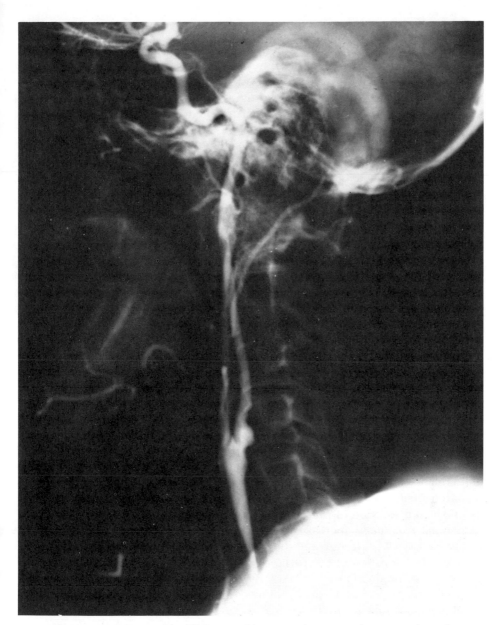

Figure 3-1. *Angiogram of left carotid artery demonstrating stenosis and a large ulcerated placque involving the internal carotid just beyond the bifurcation of the common carotid artery.*

Hemorrhage

Bleeding directly into the cerebral tissues, when the result of vascular disease, is most often associated with hypertension (Hier et al, 1977) but it may occur with a variety of pathologies affecting the cerebral vessels such as aneurysm, angioma, AV malformation, blood dyscrasia or arteritis. Anticoagulant therapy, often prescribed to prevent cerebral vascular occlusive disease, is acknowledged as a frequent cause of cerebral hemorrhage and, of course, can lead to aphasia. Finally, bleeding into an intracerebral neoplasm and trauma, while not strictly vascular problems, deserve emphasis as they are often an unsuspected and, therefore, treacherous cause of intracranial hemorrhage.

The exact pathology produced by cerebral vascular disorders varies considerably. Both thrombosis and embolism cause acute ischemia in the tissues receiving their vascular supply from the occluded vessel which, in turn, produces an area of cell death (infarct). Both neurons and the myelinated pathways are affected but the white matter is considerably less sensitive to ischemia than grey matter. The center of an infarct will be totally destroyed, but towards the periphery there may be preservation of white matter pathways and there is often a surrounding zone of lesser ischemia in which cells cease to function but cell death does not occur. In time, some of these injured neurons recuperate sufficiently to resume function and many white matter pathways survive to carry impulses again. This delayed return to function of an infarct provides one explanation (but not the only one) of the spontaneous recovery so prevalent in aphasia. The final product of vascular disease affecting the brain is the infarct, a cyst from which both neurons and white matter have disappeared, surrounded by a scarred, sclerotic zone of glia (see Fig. 3-2). Hemorrhages usually involve deeper structures and produce changes both by local destruction and by the pressure a mass lesion imposes on surrounding tissues. Initially, a hemorrhage is a large mass of blood encapsulated by compressed cerebral tissue, called a hematoma (see Fig. 3-3). The hematoma acts as a mass lesion and is the cause of maximal disruption of function. If the patient survives the initial insult the hematoma eventually decreases in size and nearly disappears, leaving only a cystic cavity with sclerotic and discolored walls.

The exact location of the pathology in the vascular tree may be of significance in the production of aphasic symptoms, even though distant from the area of infarction. The clinical picture will vary with thrombotic or embolic involvement of middle cerebral, anterior cerebral or posterior cerebral vessels and, most particularly, their branches. It is often postulated that emboli are more likely to affect terminal branches and thrombi the main trunks, but this adage has not been solidly substantiated. Infarction involving the borderzone territory (see Fig. 3-4) often indicates that the occlusion occurred at a distance, most often at the carotid bifurcation allowing partial but insufficient compensatory vascular supply via vessels of the circle of Willis (Romanul and Abramowitz, 1961). The depth of the pathology, whether cortical, subcortical or mixed, also depends on the site of vascular occlusion. The exact aphasic symptom picture (syndrome) will thus vary, to a considerable degree, with the

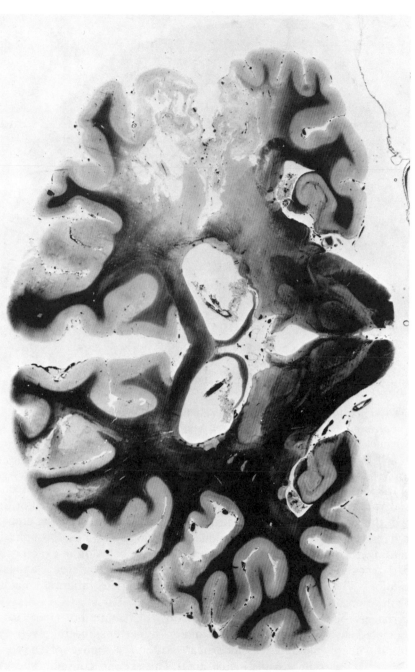

Figure 3-2. Whole brain coronal section with myelin stain demonstrating a large, old cystic infarct involving the sylvian area both above and below the sylvian fissure and extending deeply into the white matter. Note the total loss of myelinated fibers lateral to the left lateral ventricle. Clinically, the patient had the features of Wernicke aphasia.

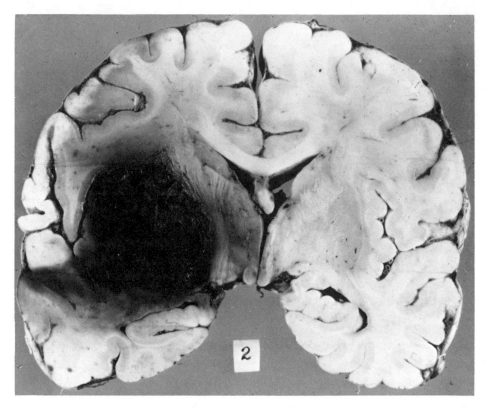

Figure 3-3. Photograph of coronal section demonstrating a massive intracerebral hemorrhage in the right hemisphere. Note destruction and distortion of
the deep nuclear centers and the surrounding area of compression and edema.

portion of the vascular tree affected. Aphasic syndromes can offer guidance to
the site and variety of vascular occlusion. The generalization suggested at the
beginning of this chapter must be kept firmly in mind, however. It is the area of
the brain damaged, not the vessel occluded, which determines the aphasic
symptomatology. Thus, two individuals with vascular occlusion in exactly the
same spot on the same vessel may present totally different aphasic
symptomatology. The area of brain infarcted can be quite different, mainly
based on variation in the collateral circulation.

Hemorrhages occur in one of two major distributions. One, most
often associated with vascular disease and/or hypertension, involves the
more central, deeply situated, subcortical structures, most often the
striatum-thalamus-internal capsule-insula area. The second common site of
hematoma, usually associated with trauma or neoplasm, involves more
superficial cortical or subcortical areas. Obviously, distinctive variation
in the aphasia characteristics will stem from the different neuroanatomical sites
of hemorrhage.

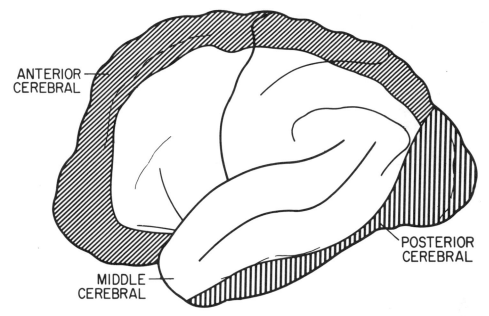

Figure 3-4. *Diagrammatic display of the territories of the three cerebral arteries over the lateral surface of the hemisphere. The central unshaded area is middle cerebral artery territory, the anterior lined area is fed by the anterior cerebral artery and the posterior lined area is fed by the posterior cerebral artery. Note that the demarcation between the territories of the individual vessels is not exact and a variable distance on either side of the suggested line is actually borderzone territory, receiving tributaries from the two contiguous supplies.*

NEOPLASM

While not noted as frequently as vascular pathology, intracranial neoplasms are certainly not uncommon as aphasia-producing lesions. Intracerebral neoplasms tend to infiltrate widely before producing focal destruction and early symptomatology from these neoplasms only rarely is sharply focal. Similarly, extracerebral but intracranial tumors (see below) usually develop slowly, allowing considerable accomodation by the cerebral tissues with only minimal disruption of function until late in the course. In fact, most early language symptoms from intracranial neoplasm can be traced directly to mass effect, most often based on interference with the cerebral blood supply or with cerebral spinal fluid circulation. The aphasia that results from early, untreated intracranial neoplasm is usually a vague, anomic disorder; rarely does it resemble one of the focal language loss syndromes to be described in Chapters 7–13. One recent study, however, demonstrated a correlation between fluent or nonfluent language disturbance and posterior or anterior locus of tumor respectively (Rosenfield and Goree, 1975), suggesting that closer evaluation of the aphasic features of early, untreated intracranial tumor might provide useful correlation information.

On the other hand, untreated tumors may produce acute, characteristic aphasia syndromes whose localization is actually distant from the site of the tumor. For instance, an intracranial tumor can produce sufficient supratentorial pressure to cause herniation of brain tissue through the tentorium. This can compromise a posterior cerebral artery (or both arteries) and if the left side is involved a syndrome of posterior involvement including alexia, agraphia, anomia and hemianopsia may result, even though the tumor is located far from the posterior cerebral territory.

In general, aphasic findings have proved to have limited value in the location of an intracranial neoplasm. In contrast, surgically treated neoplasms often yield excellent focal findings as the decompression procedure often destroys a pocket of both grey and white matter that had previously been infiltrated or compressed by the tumor. The site of surgical decompression closely resembles the cystic infarct of cerebral vascular disease, both in appearance and malfunction.

Intracranial neoplasm may be differentiated, for our purposes, into two major classes, intracerebral and extracerebral. Intracerebral neoplasms are more common as the cause of aphasia and include the glioma series (glioblastoma, astrocytoma, medulloblastoma, oligodendroglioma, ependymoma). Any variety can produce aphasia but the occurrence is variable and dependent upon both the site of the tumor and the displacement produced. With increasing age another intracerebral neoplasm, the metastasis, becomes increasingly frequent and can produce aphasia. There are many types of extracerebral tumors which, by dint of pressure, can produce language abnormality. These include meningioma, craniopharyngoma, pinealoma, acoustic neuroma, neurofibroma and a number of others. Aphasia is quite uncommon, however, as a sign of any of the extracranial tumors, and when it does occur it is almost invariably the result of distortion or displacement of cerebral tissues, often at a distance from the tumor itself. Intracerebral tumors produce language symptoms more often than extracerebral neoplasms but in neither variety does aphasia become a major complaint until late in the course of the disease.

TRAUMA

Historically trauma, particularly the brain injuries produced by war, has proved an important source of aphasic patients for academic study, and many investigators have stated that gunshot wounds to the brain offer the most accurately localized pathology available for aphasic studies (Critchley, 1970; Luria, 1970; Conrad, 1954). This statement has been challenged, however; even high velocity missile wounds produce widespread deformation of intracranial con-

tents and the more common causes of brain injury such as shrapnel, low velocity missiles and open or closed head trauma almost always cause widespread
effects on the brain. Many of the focal signs of brain trauma indicate sites which
are distant from the skull injury. Certainly, most of the head trauma seen in
civilian practice is messy, in that it injures multiple, widespread areas of the
brain. Nonetheless, with the many traffic accidents occurring these days, brain
injury is the source of a sizeable number of cases of aphasia (Levin and
Grossman, 1978). Complex nonaphasic, neurobehavioral abnormalities are almost the rule in cases of traumatic aphasia (see Ch. 16) and complicate the
problem of aphasia evaluation immensely. While the occurrence is frequent,
most cases of traumatic aphasia seen in contemporary practice do not provide
good material for the study of classic aphasic syndromes.

In addition to the actual damage done to cerebral structures by the missiles,
brain contusion or laceration, two frequent complications of trauma may play
an additional role in aphasia production. These are the traumatic intracerebral
hematomas and the extracerebral (subdural or epidural) hematomas. Extracerebral hematomas usually produce symptoms of pressure; aphasia is comparatively rare and, when present, is often only a minor symptom. Aphasia can
be noted, however, particularly as a mild word-finding disturbance in chronic
subdural hematomas; the presence of aphasia does not exclude the possibility
of an acute subdural hematoma and deserves recognition as an important variety of pathology. In contrast, traumatic intracerebral hematomas frequently
occur just below the cortical surface and, if critically located, can be the source
of specific aphasic syndromes. The degree of trauma may have been mild, and
the incident may even have been forgotten; traumatic intracerebral hematoma
deserves consideration in the evaluation of aphasia. While not frequent,
hematomas can produce clear cut aphasic syndromes.

INFECTION

Most varieties of intracranial infection produce rather widespread
neurologic symptomatology and any resulting language disorder is liable to be
lost amongst other dysfunctions. Occasionally, however, a significant aphasia
can be traced to CNS infection. By far the most common infection currently
giving rise to clear cut aphasia syndromes is herpes simplex encephalitis. While
the original symptomatology in this disorder is often widespread, with partial
clearing of the acute symptomatology, many individuals with herpes encephalitis show a severe anomia which can be retained as a long-term residual.
The anomia, however, is almost always overshadowed by a serious amnesia
(inability to learn new material). The patient may complain of memory problems when describing the inability to ''remember'' names but, with appropriate
testing, a serious defect in the learning of new material can usually be demonstrated. With ongoing recovery the common course is for greater improvement
of the word-finding problem than for the amnesia. Aphasia, therefore, is almost

never the most severe or disabling symptom of recovering herpes encephalitis but it can be demonstrated in many cases. Other types of encephalitis and/or meningitis may also on occasion lead to aphasia, but they are almost invariably accompanied by other significant neurobehavioral problems.

One notable exception is the intracranial abscess. In a manner similar to other types of intracranial tumors, an abscess can produce symptoms by pressure and by distortion of the vascular supply or the flow of CSF. Following treatment, particularly if surgically drained, a residual aphasia may persist. Cerebral abscess is relatively uncommon at present and aphasia resulting from abscess formation is certainly not frequent in clinical practice. In the preantibiotic era, however, temporal lobe abscess secondary to chronic ear infection was a frequent source of aphasia; similar syndromes are occasionally encountered in modern practice.

OTHER NEUROPATHOLOGICAL SOURCES OF APHASIA

Aphasia is occasionally seen with other varieties of intracerebral pathology but, again, most often in the company of many other neurologic and neurobehavioral dysfunctions. Multiple sclerosis only rarely causes aphasia (see Ch. 9), and when it does the aphasia is most often restricted to a problem in word-finding, almost always in combination with severe amnesia and/or dementia. Similarly, Huntington's chorea and Schilder's disease can both produce aphasia as part of their complicated clinical pictures but rarely does the language disorder reach a significant degree in contrast to other neurobehavioral symptomatology. In fact, the absence of significant aphasia in a patient with severe organic mental problems is considered a major diagnostic finding in Huntington's chorea (McHugh and Folstein, 1975). Aphasia is so mild that it often is overlooked among the multiple signs and symptoms noted in these disease states.

Finally, aphasic symptoms are commonly seen in degenerative disorders such as Alzheimer's and Pick's diseases, in slow virus infections such as Creutzfeldt-Jakob and other disorders affecting intracerebral structures. While the degree of language dysfunction may be considerable (in fact there may be a total loss of language competency in the advanced stages of these disorders) there are so many other behaviorial and neurologic problems that individuals with these disorders never present a problem of aphasia diagnosis nor is their language symptomatology useful for language research purposes.

In summary, most cases of aphasia seen in the peacetime practice of neurology arise from vascular disease with smaller numbers of clear cut cases following neoplasm or trauma. Many other intracerebral structural abnormalities may lead to language disturbance, but almost invariably the aphasia is buried among many other serious behavioral disabilities. The variety of aphasic symptoms is dependent, not upon the type of pathology, but on the location of the causative lesion. For the nonphysician aphasiologist the type of pathology underlying a case of aphasia is of limited interest. For the neurologist, however, the treatment and prognosis of an individual with aphasia is more closely linked to the variety of the pathology than to any language feature and the cause of the aphasia must be determined as accurately as possible to provide optimal treatment. There is a specific neuropathology underlying every case of aphasia and from the viewpoint of the neurologist (and the patient) the subject is of major importance.

4

Methods of Aphasia-Testing

Another reflection of the many different approaches to aphasia can be seen from the wide variety of methods used for evaluation. One would anticipate that language-testing techniques in general would show considerable similarity, or would be stereotyped and identical; this is not so. In fact, not only do standard testing techniques vary considerably but each major academic approach to language disturbance has introduced its own unique set of test methods, providing additional "chaos" to the picture of aphasia. Three different approaches to language evaluation will be discussed here. The first will outline the approach of the physician who evaluates language as part of an overall physical and mental status examination ("bedside testing"). Next, a number of the more widely used standardized aphasia test batteries will be described, and finally a brief overview will be given of the countless experimental techniques that have been created by academic specialists to probe language function. While there is some degree of overlap in the testing methods to be described, numerous and significant differences are readily apparent.

CLINICAL TESTING FOR APHASIA

Clinical testing for aphasia is the oldest, although not necessarily the best established, of the testing methods. It is less exacting and less complete and is most often performed by evaluating a few fixed language functions (i.e. naming, reading). Unfortunately, most of the functions that are tested were selected over a century ago and reflect simplified and, in some instances, obsolete concepts of language function. The traditional bedside approach is still widely used, however, and remains the most important technique available to the neurologist evaluating a patient with aphasia and so will be presented here in some detail.

Conversational Speech

Evaluation of aphasia traditionally begins with the monitoring of spontaneous or conversational verbalizations made by the patient. While many clinicians merely list descriptive features of aphasic output, many others have suggested classifying the output in two subtypes, most often called fluent or nonfluent. This dichotomy was clearly described as early as 1868 by Jackson

(1932) and the terms *fluent* and *nonfluent* were suggested by Wernicke (1908). These terms are not truly descriptive, however, and may prove misleading for the inexperienced examiner. In recent years, a number of formal studies have been performed probing the validity of this dichotomy. Each study outlined a number of specific output criteria, noted frequent combinations of output features and correlated these combinations with the anatomical locus of causative pathology. In general the early observations have been supported (Benson, 1967; Poeck, Kerschensteiner and Hartje, 1972; Wagenaar, Snow and Prins, 1975).

Nonfluent aphasic output has a number of striking characteristics. One notable feature is *decreased output,* often fewer than 10 words per minute. Actually, almost any output of less than 50 words per minute will appear abnormally sparse and appears nonfluent. A second distinct feature is *increased effort.* When attempting to produce a word, the nonfluent aphasic struggles visibly, utilizing facial grimaces, body posturing, deep breathing, hand gestures and so forth in attempts to aid output. A third characteristic is *dysarthria:* when the sounds are finally produced they are often poorly articulated and difficult to understand. A quick test for whether a sound can be considered dysarthric is for the examiner to imitate the sound produced by the patient. Dysarthric pronunciation is extremely difficult, if not impossible, for the normal speaker to imitate, as it contains sounds which are not part of the well-rehearsed group of phonemes used by normal speakers. A fourth characteristic of nonfluent speech is *decreased phrase length* (Goodglass, Quadfasel and Timberlake, 1964). Most responses by a nonfluent aphasic are limited to a single word, and even with recovery the phrase length remains notably short. The combination of features just described produces a notably unmelodic, dysrhythmic output that has been called *dysprosody* (Monrad-Krohn, 1947) and amounts to a fifth distinctive feature. Actually, the study by Goodglass et al (1964) found abnormality of speech melody to be the single most distinctive feature differentiating nonfluent from fluent aphasia. Not all of these features need to be present for an aphasic to be considered nonfluent but sparse output, short phrase length and nonmelodic speech are almost universally present in this state. One additional feature of nonfluent speech is noteworthy. Even though very few words are produced by the nonfluent aphasic, the output often conveys considerable information. The words produced are usually nouns, action verbs or descriptive adjectives, words that convey much of the information of a sentence. In contrast, there is a real decrease (almost an absence) in syntactical (grammatical, functor, filler) words except for those that are part of a short stereotyped phrase uttered as a single unit. The nonfluent aphasic patient can often communicate considerable information despite limitation of verbal production to one-word sentences or "telegraphic speech." This striking alteration of normal grammatical sentence structure has been called *agrammatism* which, in addition to deletion of syntactic language structures (prepositions, articles, adverbs, many adjectives and verbs), includes marked difficulty in handling relational words (big-small, nearer-farther), plurals, pronouns, possessives and the tense of verbs (Goodglass and Berko, 1960). Recent investigations have demonstrated that patients with nonfluent output typically have difficulty comprehending relational structures also (Samuels and Benson, 1979).

When most profound, nonfluent output may be limited to a single word or syllable ("goodbye," "Jesus Christ," "zu-zu," "ba-ba"), a condition which has been called *verbal stereotypy* (Alajouanine, 1956). While the variations in nonfluent aphasic output are vast, ranging from an isolated utterance to a subtle form of agrammatism, the features are clearly distinguishable from those seen with fluent aphasia.

The other type of output, fluent aphasia, has features that are almost the direct opposite of nonfluent aphasia. The quantity of verbal output ranges from low-normal to super-normal levels. Thus, some fluent aphasics have been transcribed with output of over 200 words per minute and most are within the normal range (100–150 words per minute) (Howes and Geschwind, 1964). Speech production in fluent aphasia demands little or no effort and articulation is normal. Similarly, phrases are of normal length, averaging about 5 words per phrase and there is a normal, acceptable melodic quality. Several characteristics of fluent output are distinctly abnormal. For one, pauses occur frequently and are qualitatively distinct from the pauses seen between each word of the nonfluent aphasic. The fluent aphasic articulates a series of words easily but tends to pause when a specific, meaningful word is needed. The word may not be readily available, and following a pause, substitution of a descriptive phrase may be attempted. The description may also depend upon a word that is unavailable, necessitating yet another description; this circling around the subject produces a wordy but meaningless output called *circumlocution*. The fluent patient may substitute a generalization (it, thing, them, etc.) for an unavailable word or merely continue without the word. Many fluent aphasics produce long sentences which contain so few substantive words that almost no information is conveyed, an output that can be called "empty speech." The pauses, then, reflect and are a product of a second distinguishing characteristic of fluent aphasic output, a deficiency of the substantive, meaningful words that make up most of nonfluent output. The production of many words that convey little information is a significant characteristic of fluent aphasia. In addition, some fluent aphasics make errors in the use of grammatical structures using incorrect verb tenses, inappropriate conditional clauses or prepositional phrases, a condition termed *paragrammatism*. This feature is not common, however, and is not present in most fluent aphasics.

One additional feature of fluent aphasia deserves strong emphasis, the occurrence of *paraphasia*. Paraphasia may be defined as a substitution within language; this may be a substitution of a syllable (called literal paraphasia or phonemic substitution), substitution of a word (verbal paraphasia, semantic substitution) or substitution of a meaningless, nonsense word (neologism). For example, a patient may introduce his wife by saying "this is my wafe," a literal paraphasic error; "this is my mother," a verbal paraphasia or "this is my bask," a neologism. Phonemic substitutions also occur in nonfluent aphasia (Blumstein, 1973) but only in a substrate of poorly articulated output. The paraphasias of nonfluent aphasia resemble (and often are) articulatory problems in contrast to the paraphasia of fluent output which appears to involve true substitutions. While some posterior aphasics may be aware of some of their paraphasias, they are usually unaware of most of the substitutions. When an aphasic has a rapid verbal output, liberally laced with paraphasic substitutions, the verbalization becomes incomprehensible and has been termed *jargon aphasia*.

Utilizing these output characteristics, the clinical studies demonstrate that the verbalizations of most aphasics fall into one of the two subtypes, fluent or nonfluent. In addition, a clear cut anatomical correlation for the two varieties of verbal output has been described for over a century and confirmed by extensive clinical investigations (see Ch. 15 for additional details of the neuroanatomical correlation of aphasic output).

Repetition

The ability to repeat, exactly, the words presented by the examiner is a significant language function that, until recently, has not received sufficient attention. Repetition is comparatively easy to test at the bedside and can usually be judged on a simple pass/fail scale. Starting with simple tasks such as repeating digits (one, twenty-six, three seventy-four and so on) and frequently-used words (house, automobile), the complexity of the repetition tasks can be increased to the level of complex sentences ("When the tired businessman returned home he found the house filled with his son's friends."), multisyllabic words ("constitution," "Congressional Investigating Committee"), and phrases featuring multiple relationships and complex syntactic structures ("when he gets here we can ask him if he put it there"). Many aphasic patients have tremendous difficulty repeating exactly what is said, even at an elementary level. The difficulty often reflects, rather accurately, problems of verbal output or comprehension of spoken language but some aphasic individuals have problems of repetition that are considerably greater than either (see Ch. 7).

In sharp contrast, some aphasics are unexpectedly good at repeating what the examiner has said, despite notable abnormalities in spontaneous output, comprehension or both. A strong, almost mandatory, tendency to repeat what has just been said by the examiner is called *echolalia* and, when present, is of considerable diagnostic significance (see Ch. 8). Fully developed echolalia encompasses entire phrases and sentences. The echoed phrase may be the only output the patient can offer. In other cases, the echoed phrase may be followed by a run of jargon output with the patient apparently unaware of what he is saying. Most patients with echolalia show the completion phenomenon (Stengel, 1947); thus, if started on a phrase which is not completed (red, white and ____), the correct word will be supplied automatically. Even more dramatic is the ability of some of these aphasic patients to continue poems or nursery rhymes initiated by the examiner. *Echoing* is often considered a similar phenomenon but it is clearly a separate disturbance. In this state the aphasic patient repeats a single word or a short phrase uttered by the examiner, often inflected as a question and almost invariably indicating a need to reinforce a poorly understood bit of language. Echoing is seen most frequently in cases of aphasia with auditory comprehension difficulties. A similar phenomenon is a well-known characteristic of the deaf.

Comprehension of Spoken Language

The ability to comprehend what is said has proved to be the most difficult language function to test adequately. Both bedside clinical evaluations and formal, standardized tests of language comprehension may prove difficult and, not infrequently, produce misleading results. A classic method for probing comprehension has been to monitor the patient's response to verbally presented commands. The ability to carry out complex commands, particularly when several unrelated motor actions must be performed in sequence, indicates a considerable degree of intact comprehension in an aphasic patient. On the other hand, failure to carry out commands under these circumstances does not necessarily indicate serious comprehension difficulties, and there are conditions where aphasic patients will carry out certain verbal commands when they can comprehend no other spoken or written language. Thus the response to verbal commands is easily misinterpreted. Both apraxia (disturbance in the ability to carry out motor activities on verbal command) and difficulty in maintaining sequences can seriously interfere with motor performance tasks and yet not prove that the patient has specific language comprehension difficulties. To obviate problems in motor responses, tests which require only minimal motor movement, such as yes/no questions, can be used. Unfortunately, some aphasics cannot handle the movements for yes and no, producing undecipherable, perseverative or combined responses and the examiner cannot be certain whether the response indicates success or failure of comprehension. Another approach demanding only limited motor activity requests that the patient point to objects about the room or in an array placed in front of him when the examiner gives the name of the object. If the patient can successfully accomplish the task of pointing to a named object, the request can be made increasingly complex by offering vague functional descriptions of the same objects or by demanding that a series of objects be pointed out in the exact sequence given by the examiner. Even the motor task of pointing, however, is failed by some aphasic patients with severe motor problems and this failure may inaccurately exaggerate the patient's problems in comprehension.

Comprehension is rarely an all-or-none phenomenon. Some aphasic patients comprehend frequently used words, but fail to understand low frequency words. Others comprehend concrete, meaningful, real-world names, but fail to understand relational or syntactical structures such as prepositions, possessives, verb tenses, etc. Some aphasics comprehend individual words readily but fail to understand the same word when part of a sequence (e.g. they correctly point to the door, window and floor when presented individually but fail when asked to point to the same three in sequence) (Albert, 1972). There is much yet to be learned about comprehension of spoken language and its testing, but it is almost never correct to state that comprehension is either absent or normal in aphasia. Most aphasics can understand some language and, conversely, almost all have at least some problems with comprehension. At present, abnormalities of language comprehension should be described as accurately as possible in both qualitative and quantitative terms. In the end, a good rule to remember is that most aphasics comprehend more than the testing indicates.

Word-Finding

Almost without exception, all aphasics show some degree of difficulty in word-finding, although the degree and circumstances vary considerably. Aphasic word-finding problems have been given many different names; the commonly used term, *anomia,* will be used here.

Testing for word-finding is comparatively easy. Items can be demonstrated and the patient asked to give their name; failure to produce the name indicates a word-finding problem. Many examiners follow a failure to name by offering a multiple choice list of names including the correct one; this is *not* a test of naming, however. Rather, this represents a test of auditory comprehension; unfortunately, success at this task is frequently misinterpreted to indicate that the patient actually does "know" the name of the object. It is better to follow the patient's failure to produce a name by prompting (offering a cue). The initial phoneme càn be presented (phonetic prompting) or an open-ended sentence given in which the missing word would be the appropriate ending (contextual prompting, "You write with a _____.").

Word-finding ability is important in evaluating aphasia and word-finding tests should be included in all examinations of aphasia. A recent study of the varieties of anomia (Benson, 1979) suggested eight tests for word-finding that could be performed informally and that offered useful diagnostic information. These included:

1. auditing conversational speech for word-finding problems to determine whether the defect stems from word production problems (faulty articulation, paraphasia) or an inability to retrieve the correct word;

2. testing the ability to name items by visual presentation from the following categories: objects, parts of objects, body parts, colors, geometric shapes, numerals, letters and actions;

3. testing the ability to name items on tactile presentation;

4. testing the ability to name from auditory stimulation;

5. testing the ability to name illness-oriented items;

6. testing the ability to name objects from a verbal description of their function;

7. monitoring the ability to benefit from cues (prompting) when naming is failed;

8. testing the ability to produce lists of words from a given category (animals, articles of furniture, words beginning with the letter "R," etc.).

By utilizing these tests and neighborhood neurologic and aphasic signs, a number of distinct varieties of anomia can be postulated and a neuroanatomical correlation suggested for each variation (see Ch. 15).

It must be remembered that a number of "nonaphasic" cerebral abnormalities such as dementia, confusional states and others also produce notable problems in word-finding. Word-finding difficulty is not an exclusive indication of aphasia. When anomia is present, however, aphasia must be seriously considered and the responses to word-finding tests may prove helpful in establishing the appropriate diagnosis.

Reading

Loss of the ability to read following brain damage (alexia), either with or without accompanying aphasia, has been recognized for centuries and reading is comparatively easy to evaluate, at least in a gross manner. When quantified results are required, however, standardized test material will be necessary. Simply offering the written name of a body part or room object for the patient to identify is an easy reading test to perform at the bedside. If the patient is successful at this level, more difficult written material including phrases or sentences, dependent on low frequency or relational types of words, can be presented for interpretation. An even more challenging bedside test of reading ability is to request understanding of paragraph-length material from a newspaper or magazine. A simple determination of the retention of reading comprehension is to request that the aphasic patient recognize words spelled aloud by the examiner (Geschwind, 1962; Howes, 1962). While not always accurate, most patients with parietal-temporal alexia fail to recognize words spelled aloud, while those with occipital alexia perform quite well (see Ch. 11 for details). The most common error made in the testing of reading ability is equating the ability to read out loud with the ability to comprehend written material. Many aphasics with verbal output disturbances fail when asked to read aloud but some of them comprehend written material adequately. The opposite can also be seen, aphasic patients who read aloud flawlessly but in whom comprehension of what has been read cannot be demonstrated. It is the ability to comprehend written language that is to be monitored; it is the loss of this ability that is called *alexia*. Alexia will be further discussed in Chapter 11.

Writing

Almost without exception, every aphasic suffers some difficulty in writing (*agraphia*). An initial test is to request that the patient write his own name. Some aphasics fail even this most elementary test, but many succeed and it must be recognized that the ability to sign one's name is sufficiently over-learned that many aphasics with severe writing disturbance produce their own signature readily even when they cannot write any other words. Testing of writing ability, therefore, should not stop at the level of the patient's signature. Writing tests should include the ability to write words and sentences to dictation and to produce written sentences to command (i.e., describe your job). In nonhemiplegic patients, writing should be tested in each hand. Comparison can be made of the ability to copy written material with the ability to produce similar words to dictation. There are qualitative variations in agraphia and four aspects of writing disorder deserve specific attention: 1) defects of the mechanics of handwriting (orthography); 2) abnormalities of written syntax; 3) disorders of semantic content and 4) an inability to spell. Unfortunately, the variations of writing disorders that can follow brain damage combined with marked premorbid individual variations have defied demonstration of exact clinical-anatomical correlations of agraphia. At present, tests of writing ability are primarily used as screening devices for language disturbance, but in the future variations in agraphia should come to have considerable meaning for the student of language problems.

In summary, the clinical testing of aphasia is inexact, nonstandardized and constantly being altered. Therein lies both the weakness and the strength of the clinical approach. Many of the techniques utilized in the formal aphasia batteries and in the research tests of language dysfunction were derived from the experiences gained in the clinic or at the bedside. An experienced examiner can perform a clinical evaluation on an aphasic patient's language in only a few minutes and, by focusing on the primary problem, obtain an in-depth view of the type of aphasia that is often more accurate and exacting than that available from either the formal aphasia batteries or the most advanced research techniques. However, even in the best hands, the results of clinical testing are subject to theoretical biases and in the hands of inexperienced examiners the clinical evaulation can prove disastrously misleading. The need for more exact, standardized testing techniques is obvious.

FORMAL TESTS OF APHASIA

Following the lead of Henry Head (1926), Weisenburg and McBride (1935) produced a battery of tests to define the language qualities of aphasic patients. While never widely used, this battery was the harbinger of a new era in aphasia assessment. In the past 25 years a large number of formal test batteries have been devised for the assessment of aphasia, standardized to a greater or lesser degree and utilized widely. While there is considerable overall similarity in the tests, there are also a number of significant differences. Thers is no consensus as to which battery or batteries are best and all of the tests to be mentioned are favored and in use somewhere at the present time. Almost every aphasic entering a formal aphasia therapy program is given part or all of one or more of these tests and the results from the tests are widely used in both research projects and clinical reports. This section will list some of the currently popular tests along with some of their more distinctive characteristics. The test batteries will not be outlined in full detail; readers desiring such information are referred to the references given for each test battery.

One of the earliest tests and one still in wide use is Eisenson's *Examining for Aphasia* (1954). This is a medium-length test, divided into two functional sections, expressive and receptive; many of the techniques of language evaluation presented in this test are also found in the later tests. Of a similar nature and also among the early test batteries is the *Sklar Aphasia Scale* (1966) which covers a broad inventory of language functions. While use of the Sklar test has not been widespread and use of the Eisenson test is decreasing, both remain the major testing technique used in some centers.

Subsequently, two long and rationally formulated aphasia tests came into fairly general use. *The Language Modalities Test for Aphasia* of Wepman (1961) and *The Minnesota Test for the Differential Diagnosis of Aphasia* of Schuell (1957) were presented for general use at about the same time but have significant differences in composition. The Schuell test is specifically designed to classify aphasic patients into one of five categories that indicate the prognosis for language recovery and offers an extensive evaluation of many separate language functions. The entire test is both long and difficult to present but provides a great deal of information about the aphasic's language dysfunction. On the other hand, the Wepman test was designed along basic psychological parameters, emphasizing the specific stimulus given and the response obtained. Both the Wepman and the Schuell tests have subsections that have proved valuable for evaluating aphasic disturbances. There has been a strong tendency for aphasia therapists to utilize subsections of both tests, particularly portions of the Schuell test, either in isolation or in combination with sections of other test batteries. It is worth noting that while the Schuell test was devised by an aphasia therapist to guide therapists in planning treatment, and the Wepman test was devised by a psychologist and emphasizes psychological characteristics, the findings from the Wepman test have proved helpful to the aphasia therapist and the Schuell test has been used extensively in psychological research programs.

In more recent years, a comparatively simple and eminently quantifiable test of language disability, *The Porch Index of Communicative Ability* (PICA) (1967), has become popular. The PICA takes less time to administer than many of the aphasia batteries mentioned (approximately one hour) and can be repeated with excellent test-retest reliability. While easier to administer, the scoring system is exacting and demands thorough training and great care. The PICA offers excellent quantitative results but comparatively little qualitative information. For instance, there is little evaluation of spontaneous or conversational speaking, limited testing of praxis and little recognition of complicating factors such as the Gerstmann syndrome. The greatest usefulness of the PICA appears to lie in recording language recovery after onset of aphasia. It has been claimed that the prognosis of a given case of aphasia can be predicted from the original PICA score and the recovery monitored by repeated administrations of the test. Unfortunately, therapy directed toward tasks used on the PICA itself can improve the score without truly altering functional use of language. This trap is easily avoided, however, and the PICA has attained significant status among current testing techniques.

In recent years, a number of additional tests have been introduced and attained some popularity. The most widely used of these later tests is the

Boston Diagnostic Aphasia Evaluation (BDAE) (Goodglass and Kaplan, 1972), which provides the widest range of evaluation techniques but is so lengthy that it must be administered in separate sessions over the course of several days. The results of BDAE testing can be difficult to interpret as they demand knowledge of a system of aphasic syndromes that is neither widely known nor totally accepted (see Ch. 6). The BDAE is considerably more inclusive than any of the previously described tests, however, and when properly interpreted offers far more diagnostic information. A shorter language test, based on the BDAE, is called the *Western Aphasia Battery* (Kertesz and Poole, 1974), and is used in several Canadian centers. Another closely related aphasia battery that has been used more extensively for research is the *Neurosensory Center Test for Aphasia* (NSCTA) (Spreen and Benton, 1960). Excellent normal values (percentiles) are available for individual subtests on the NSCTA and each subtest can be rated separately or the language disturbance rated in its entirety. Both the BDAE and the NSCTA are superior to previous tests for diagnostic purposes and as research tools, but to date neither has proved superior for the therapist planning a rehabilitation program.

Finally, there are several tests available that measure the ability to communicate in general rather than monitoring specific language dysfunction. The original example, and still a widely used test, is the *Functional Communication Profile* (FCP) devised by Taylor (1968). There is comparatively little quantification as this test relies on comparative observations by the evaluator. The observations are easily classed, even by untrained personnel, and formal evaluations have demonstrated good inter-observer reliability. The FCP is not a standardized test but has proved useful in making qualitative judgments and evaluating rapid changes in communication. At the present time another, more complete evaluation of communication ability is under study. This is the *Assessment of Communicative Activities Relevant to Daily Living* devised by Holland and colleagues (1977) under contract from the National Institutes of Health. So far this communication scale has not been offered for general use, but upon completion of the study it should become generally available.

In summary, a fairly large number of distinctively different formal tests of aphasia are presently being administered. Each test has proved useful in some phase of aphasia evaluation and no single test has proved clearly superior to all others. Inasmuch as one major function of the formal aphasia batteries is to guide the therapist in planning rehabilitation, the choice of test remains an individual decision, each therapist utilizing the battery that best serves his or her particular needs. The field of test batteries will probably narrow in the future, but with aphasia therapy still in an early formative stage there is an obvious need for continued experimentation and improvement of the aphasia assessment techniques.

RESEARCH TESTING PROCEDURES

Most of the radical changes in the approach to aphasia evaluation seen in the past several decades stem from the use of psychological experimentation techniques. Dating from the pioneering efforts of Head (1926) and Weisenburg and McBride (1935) the utilization of psychological testing techniques to delineate language abnormality has expanded greatly. Current activity is sufficiently great to warrant publication of three specialty journals, either exclusively or primarily devoted to the study of language malfunction and, in addition, many articles on this topic spill over into other scientific and academic journals and many books on studies of language dysfunction appear annually. Even a cursory review of this plethora of language research material extends far beyond the scope of this volume and only a few of the more prominent approaches can be highlighted.

Psychological approaches to language (usually called neuropsychology and differentiated from the linguistic approach to psychology known as psycholinguistics) have only a short background as measured in years but have been brilliantly performed by many outstanding investigators. These include reknowned leaders in the field such as Luria, Hecaen, Zangwill, Goodglass and Benton and their co-workers who have produced innumerable advances through controlled study of language impairments. DeRenzi and Vignolo of Italy are best known for their Token Test (1962), considered an excellent probe of subtle comprehension difficulties. Leading American investigators include Goodglass, Benton and Teuber whose output includes many studies of language and language-related disorders, performed with excellent, replicable scientific design. The number of psychologists and linguists currently studying language disorders is enormous and the neuropsychological study of language appears to rank among the most actively advancing of all fields of knowledge at present.

The investigation of aphasia by linguists, or psychologists with training and experience in linguistics, started somewhat later than the initial neuropsychological studies. The psycholinguistic approach combines a background knowledge of linguistics with the scientific design of psychology. Some psycholinguists specialize in phonological problems, others in syntactical or grammatical functions and others have investigated semantic processes. Much of the early work by linguists, however, was centered on normal language and only recently have linguists discovered the wealth of information available from disordered language and started to utilize aphasic patients as research subjects. Most psycholinguistic studies are still designed to probe normal language function by studying aphasic disability; the potential for the reciprocal action, an improved understanding of aphasia, is obvious. Both neuropsychologic and psycholinguistic approaches have produced valuable results, some of which will be listed briefly, but this short review represents only a superficial glimpse of the rich body of work currently being performed.

Abnormalities of syntax have been investigated in the aphasic. Goodglass and Berko (1960) demonstrated consistent defects in the syntactical structure of the output of certain aphasics, a state which has been called *agrammatism*. Agrammatic output is characterized by a tendency to omit relational language words, articles, prepositions, conjunctions and minor modifiers, and is one of the most consistent features of nonfluent aphasia. Recent studies (Zurif, Caramazza and Myerson, 1972) suggest that comparable comprehension defects, an inability to "understand" these relational words, often coexists with agrammatic output. These individuals handle (verbalize and comprehend) substantive, semantically significant words far better than the relational, syntactically significant words. Correlation of these studies with the neuroanatomy of aphasia demonstrates that disability in handling syntactical processes occurs with Broca or other anterior aphasia and implies, strongly, that grammatical performance is dependent on intact frontal language functions.

Intelligence in aphasia (whether retained or lost) has been widely but rather futilely debated. Disturbed language function invalidates most of the recognized techniques of intelligence assessment. To some observers this is evidence of decreased intelligence (Goldstein, 1948; Bay, 1962) but others believe that some aphasics retain normal or nearly normal intelligence which is locked in by the language problem (Kennedy and Wolf, 1936; Orgass et al, 1972). Nonverbal tests such as the Ravens Matrices (Ravens, 1952) and the performance section of the Wechsler Adult Intelligence Score (Wechsler, 1958) have been used as substitute techniques for gauging retained intelligence in aphasia but demand a great deal of unsatisfactory interpolation. The crux of the controversy, of course, centers on disagreement over the definition of intelligence and most current discussions flounder on the vexed question of what constitutes intelligence (Piercy, 1964). It is safe to say that most aphasics have more understanding and more intelligence than can be demonstrated by present evaluation techniques (Zangwill, 1969) but this certainly does not imply that intelligence is normal in all aphasics. Hecaen and Albert (1978) note the frequent association of impaired intelligence (on nonverbal tasks) with impaired auditory comprehension and/or semantic paraphasia, suggesting a relationship between Wernicke aphasia and defective intelligence. The constancy of this correlation can be questioned, however, leaving the exact relationship of defective intellectual ability and language dysfunction unsettled (Hoops and Lebrun, 1974). Hopefully, improved neuropsychological techniques of the future will overcome part of the dilemma and provide better gauges of the residual intelligence in aphasia.

Another long-studied facet, the relationships of aphasia to cerebral dominance, handedness and the functional laterality of the hemispheres, is also under active investigation. The unique role of the left hemisphere for language was recognized by Broca as early as 1865 and some claim that Dax had presented this correlation even earlier (Benton, 1964). Subsequent clinical observations have suggested that similar asymmetries of hemispheric functions influence a number of mental activities (Gloning, 1969; Warrington, 1969; Bogen and Bogen, 1969; Gainotti, 1972; Galin, 1974). Language dysfunction has been studied following section of the corpus callosum (Geschwind and Kaplan, 1962; Gazzaniga and Sperry, 1967), following hemispherectomy (Smith and Sugar, 1975), after intracarotid barbiturate injection (Wada and Rasmussen, 1960; Wildmore et al, 1978), and after asymmetrical interference by dichotic auditory stimulation (Broadbent, 1971; Kimura, 1967; Sparks and Geschwind, 1968). Neuroanatomical asymmetry of the two hemispheres (Geschwind ' and Levitsky, 1968; Yakovlev and Rakic, 1966; Galaburda et al, 1978) has also been demonstrated. Technical improvements have provided better knowledge of the respective hemisphere's role in language and related function but the field is immense, much remains uncertain and unexplained and the field of investigation is extremely active at present.

Dichotic listening techniques have been used extensively in recent years to study both language function and malfunction. The simultaneous presentation of different verbal or nonverbal messages to each ear and, hypothetically, to the contralateral hemispheres, following Broadbent's original description (1971), was used by Kimura and co-workers to study language dominance (1967). The technique has been used by many other investigators to study individual linguistic functions (Bryden, 1963; Shankweiler and Studdert-Kennedy, 1967; Spellacy, 1970) and remains an active research tool for both linguistics and neuropsychology.

Finally, psycholinguists and linguists have produced elegant studies of the characteristics of aphasic output. These studies include outlines of the phonology of aphasic output, particularly the articulatory disturbances of anterior aphasia (LeCours and Lhermitte, 1969; Blumstein, 1973), detailed descriptions of disturbances in semantic function (Osgood, 1957; Goodglass and Baker, 1976) and demonstration of abnormalities in syntactical relationships in aphasia (Zurif, Caramazza and Myerson, 1972; Goodglass et al, 1972).

Both the neuropsychologic and the linguistic research approaches to aphasia are extremely active, cover a broad range of topics and are changing rapidly at present. It will probably take at least a decade before this interrelated activity can jell sufficiently to allow a consensus to be formed as to the more important discoveries. Several recent books (Goodglass and Blumstein, 1973; Whitaker and Whitaker, 1976a, 1976b, 1977, 1979) and the journals *Brain and Language, Cortex* and *Neuropsychologia* are recommended as resources for current information in the fast-moving field of psycholinguistics.

5

Localization of Aphasia-Producing Lesions

Since the time of Broca, neuroanatomical localization of the site of pathology underlying aphasia has been a major aspect of the study of aphasia, particularly for the neurologist-aphasiologist. Over the years, a number of different means of localizing aphasia-producing lesions have been suggested and tried but not all have been successful. In fact, localization of aphasia-producing lesions in the living patient has proved immensely difficult, and until recent technical advances it has never been more than partially successful. Traditionally, the aphasic syndromes have been outlined clinically and then correlated with any information allowing neuroanatomical localization. All of the localizing techniques devised thus far have significant defects, but by utilizing several of them exact localizations can often be determined. The major localization techniques currently in use (and all successful methods continue to be used) will be reviewed here.

NEUROPATHOLOGICAL CORRELATIONS

The use of necropsy material is the original and remains the classic means of localizing aphasia-producing lesions. Most of the originally reported aphasia cases were described clinically and later correlated with the neuroanatomical location of pathology. The work of Broca, Wernicke, Bastian, Dejerine and many others relied heavily upon the anatomical localizations available from postmortem findings. In 1922, Henschen collected over a thousand cases of aphasia from the medical literature that had both clinical information to outline the aphasic symptoms and sufficient evidence (mostly postmortem) to allow anatomical localization. Uncounted hundreds of additional cases have been published subsequently, correlating aphasia with autopsy findings, and postmortem studies remain a major means of localizing aphasia-producing lesions.

There are a number of drawbacks to postmortem material as a means of localization, however. Most seriously, the patient must be dead before the autopsy material becomes available. Not only is this an unhappy criterion but it is imperative that the patient not have additional CNS pathology between the time of the recorded clinical examination and the time that the brain becomes available for study. For patients to develop clear cut aphasic syndromes, they must remain alive for a significant period of time. Often one or two months must pass after onset before a distinct aphasia syndrome can be outlined. Patients who remain alive through this period often continue living, in comparatively good health, for many years. Not only are they often lost to follow-up but there is constant jeopardy of additional cerebral pathology complicating or totally obviating any anatomical correlation. On the other hand, altogether too many cases reported in the literature, particularly those in the early literature, died soon after the onset of the aphasia, never having developed a clearly delineated clinical picture.

Despite these drawbacks, the use of necropsy material remains a key means of providing neuroanatomical localization for aphasia-producing lesions. Without question, the accuracy of anatomical location available from postmortem study is far more exact than that provided by any of the others to be discussed and autopsy localization will remain an important source of clinical correlations for future aphasia studies.

NEUROSURGICAL CORRELATIONS

Intracranial pathology that must be treated by surgical excision often produces aphasia. A patient treated surgically for intracranial aneurysm, A-V malformation, intracerebral hematoma, abscess or brain tumor may suffer a specific aphasia syndrome as a residual and can be studied for anatomical-clinical correlation purposes. The surgeons usually record the anatomical area involved in their surgical treatment as exactly as possible and the aphasia itself may be studied and classified long after the surgery is performed, at a time when the language syndrome is stable. Despite the interval, details of the anatomical localization will still be available for correlation purposes. A number of major studies of aphasia have utilized surgical material, the most prominent of which is the study of Hecaen and Angelergues (1964) that consists primarily of tumor and trauma cases. Postoperative neurosurgical cases can be considered good subjects for investigating the anatomical localization of aphasia.

Another major type of neurosurgical study, although based on a different approach, is exemplified by the work of Penfield and Roberts (1959), who stimulated various areas of the brain including portions of the "language area" and recorded their results. By using this focal stimulation procedure a number of important observations of language function were described.

The surgical correlation method has a number of drawbacks. Exact anatomical landmarks are often difficult for the neurosurgeon to identify because of the limited opening of the craniotomy. The amount of bone flap turned is usually as small as is practical, providing limited visibility for identification of neuroanatomical structures. This problem is frequently complicated by distortion of the brain structures in the area of the surgical field by edema, bleeding, tumor pressure or contusion; and, not infrequently, individual variation in the gyral formation obviates accurate recognition because of the limited aperture.

In addition, the prime duty of the neurosurgeon is toward the patient, not toward accurate anatomical localization, and surgeons never risk the patient's safety to better ascertain exact anatomical definitions. Also, the surgeon usually observes only the surface of the cortex and has limited information concerning the extent and effect of the pathology lying subcortically. Tumor cases infiltrate far beyond the area treated surgically, providing yet another source of inaccuracy. Many factors, therefore, decrease the positive information available from intracerebral surgical studies. Despite these limitations neurosurgical case material can be used for correlation with aphasia, often with excellent results.

POSTTRAUMATIC SKULL DEFECTS

Through the years many extensive studies recording localizing correlations of aphasia have utilized damage to the brain underlying trauma to the skull. Major studies such as that of Marie and Foix (1917), Luria (1970), Schiller (1947), Conrad (1954) and Russell and Espir (1961) utilized the site of skull damage to localize the aphasic syndrome. The procedure used is simple and relatively straightforward. As the patient is recovering from the head injury, the aphasia can be evaluated carefully; the site of damage to the skull is demonstrated readily, either by direct palpation or by the use of simple skull x-rays. Both localizing procedures are nonmorbid and provide an exact point to correlate with the aphasia findings.

There are a great many deficiencies in the use of skull defects to localize aphasia-producing pathology, however. In the first place, the site of the skull defect does not necessarily indicate the specific area of the brain injured; in fact, the external locus may be totally misleading. This is particularly true when the injury results from a low velocity missile or from shrapnel (see Ch. 3). To overcome this problem, a number of studies have attempted to trace the intracranial path of the missile using site of entrance and exit, but again tremendous variation is acknowledged. Similarly, the depth of the injury cannot be estimated from external data. At best the examiner must base a guess on the depth of damage from the extent of surface involvement but it is well-recognized that the amount of skull damage may have no correspondence or even an inverse relationship to the amount of brain damaged.

Nonetheless, some degree of localization can be ascertained by noting the site of skull penetration. Even the study of Conrad (1954), interpreted by the author as evidence against localization of aphasia-producing lesions, clearly demonstrates differences in the type of aphasia dependent on the location (anterior-posterior) of the skull defect. The more recent wars, particularly the Korea and Vietnam conflicts, have produced fewer studies localizing aphasia-producing lesions. This may be the result of differences in the type of cranial injury suffered; another possible cause appears to be improved transport which affords less opportunity to study the aphasia at the hospital where surgical treatment was performed. Correlation of aphasia symptoms with the site of skull defect has been used less frequently in recent years, and with the improved techniques of investigation now available, will probably find little use in the future.

CORRELATION WITH THE NEUROLOGIC EXAMINATION

A neurologic examination is easily done, produces no morbidity or discomfort and is routinely performed on patients with significant aphasia. The neurologic examination, therefore, is readily available for correlation with the aphasia symptomatology and offers useful correlation data. Unfortunately, the neurologic exam is often performed poorly and/or reported inadequately and there has been altogether too little attempt to correlate information from the routine exam with the aphasic syndromes. Many portions of the neurologic examination are of considerable value in helping localize the aphasia-producing lesion and some of these will be described briefly.

Visual Sensory Examination

The presence of a visual field defect often has significant localizing value. A full hemianopic field defect suggests parietal or occipital involvement, usually deep in the hemisphere involving the lateral geniculate nucleus, or, more often, the geniculo-calcarine pathways. A superior quadrantanopsia strongly suggests temporal lobe pathology (involving Meyer's loop) while the presence of an inferior quadrantanopsia usually indicates pathology involving the visual pathways deep in the parietal lobe. Unilateral visual inattention often has localizing value also. Thus, unilateral extinction to double simultaneous stimulation affecting one quadrant or one visual field often has the same localizing value as the full field defect. An important exception, however, is the unilateral inattention caused by frontal-limbic pathology (see Ch. 16) which, in itself, represents another valuable localizing finding.

Ocular Motor Functions

Oculomotor abnormalities often offer valuable localizing information, but most often the pathology is in the brain stem and is not associated with aphasia. Conjugate deviation of gaze, however, usually indicates pathology involving either the frontal or the parietal-occipital eye field in the hemisphere ipsilateral to the direction of conjugate gaze. (An uncommon exception is the pontine conjugate deviation in which the gaze is directed away from the side of the pathology.) A lesser degree of occular deviation, called gaze palsy, has also been described (Holmes, 1918). This problem involves an inability to gaze fully to one direction and suggests pathology in the opposite hemisphere. Asymmetry of optokinetic-nystagmus appears to have similar lateralizing value but most investigators doubt that more exact localization of pathology can be based on asymmetry of OKN alone.

Motor Examination

The presence of a significant motor paralysis is a finding of unquestioned value. When a spastic paralysis involves the entire side of the body (spastic hemiplegia), a deep-lying lesion involving the internal capsule or motor pathways rostral or caudal to this area can be suspected. In general a total hemiplegia with weakness involving both limbs and the face to a nearly equal degree suggests a deep lesion, while weakness of a single limb or part of a limb suggests either cortical pathology or a small discrete white matter destruction. The presence of a crural paralysis, weakness involving the leg and shoulder but not the arm or face, strongly suggests pathology in the anterior cerebral artery territory. Greater weakness of proximal in contrast to distal musculature is suggestive (but not pathognomonic) of involvement in the borderzone between the tributaries of the middle cerebral and the posterior cerebral arteries. Middle cerebral artery occulsion, on the other hand, is said to produce a predilection weakness, primarily involving the antigravity muscles (flexors of the upper extremity, extensors of the lower extremities). While not absolute, the patterns of paralysis are helpful localizers.

Sensory Examination

Excellent localizing information can often be obtained from the routine sensory evaluation. Loss of primary sensations, pain and temperature, suggest pathology deep in the CNS, usually at the level of the thalamus or lower. On the other hand, when pain responses are near normal but a distinct asymmetry of cortical sensory function can be demonstrated (such as position sense, double simultaneous stimulation, two-point discrimination, graphesthesia and stereognosis), the pathology probably involves either the parietal cortex or pathways connecting the thalamus to the parietal lobe. When aphasia is caused by cerebral vascular disease, "deep" sensory loss often suggests a large, wedgeshaped lesion, usually secondary to occlusion of branches of the middle cerebral artery near its takeoff from the internal carotid artery. Cortical sensory loss alone, when it accompanies aphasia, suggests occlusion of a distal branch of the middle cerebral artery.

The presence of a "pseudothalamic" pain syndrome may have localizing value. In this unusual pain syndrome patients show a disturbance of cortical sensory functions and, some months after the onset of sensory abnormality, begin to complain of constant pain and paresthesia in the affected limbs. The pain is not as excruciating as that usually described for the thalamic pain syndrome, and the discomfort is neither increased nor altered by manipulation or palpation of the involved limb. Nonetheless, these patients complain of considerable dysesthesia. Pseudothalamic pain syndrome associated with aphasia usually indicates pathology located in the white matter just below the parietal operculum (SII area). When pseudothalamic pain is present with aphasia it is usually in conjunction with conduction aphasia, a disorder in which the pathology often involves the white matter just deep to the supramarginal gyrus (see Ch. 7) affecting language and sensory pathways simultaneously.

Motor Praxis

The presence of ideomotor apraxia (Geschwind, 1965; Benson and Geschwind, 1971; Heilman, 1979) often proves valuable as a localizing finding. Three variations of motor apraxia consistently offer localizing information. In the type often called *parietal apraxia,* the patient has difficulty carrying out, on verbal command, activities with either the buccofacial or the limb musculature even though these activities are easily done spontaneously or on imitation. The pathology most frequently involves white matter in the anterior-inferior parietal lobe of the dominant hemisphere, most often deep to the supramarginal gyrus. A second variety, the most common type of ideomotor apraxia, has been called *sympathetic dyspraxia.* In this disorder, a patient with a right hemiplegia fails to utilize the intact left limbs to carry out verbal commands. In contrast, the ability of the left limbs to mimic movements is normal. Characteristically the pathology affects the motor association cortex of the dominant hemisphere. A third type, quite rare and sometimes called *callosal apraxia,* features a normal performance of commanded movements with the right limbs but failure to perform the same movements with the left limbs, when the movements are verbally requested. The pathology in this variation affects the anterior corpus callosum or fibres traversing this pathway. The names for these variations of ideomotor apraxia were suggested by Liepmann (1900, 1905) who also suggested the anatomical-clinical correlations. Leipmann's correlations have been verified innumerable times and the neuroanatomical localizing information available from praxis testing can be accepted with considerable confidence (see Ch. 16 for an additional description of apraxia).

Many other symptoms and/or signs can be demonstrated by the techniques of a neurobehavioral examination and many of these have considerable localizing value. Examples would include *acalculia* (Hecaen, 1962), *constructional disturbance* (Warrington, 1969), *dressing disturbance* (Brain, 1941), *visual agnosia* (Rubens and Benson, 1971), *reduplicative paramnesia* (Benson, Gardner, Meadows, 1976), *Capgras' syndrome* (Alexander, Stuss, Benson, 1979), the *Gerstmann syndrome* (Gerstmann, 1931; Benton, 1961, 1977) and many others. Each of these neurobehavioral defects has potential localizing value and many occur in conjunction with aphasia, adding to the store of neurologic data available for localizing an aphasic syndrome. A number of individual neurobehavioral problems will be discussed further in Chapter 16.

ELECTROENCEPHALOGRAPHY

An electroencephalogram is performed regularly, in many institutions routinely, on all patients who suffer cerebral damage including those with aphasia. An EEG is performed easily, has little or no morbidity and is comparatively inexpensive. The EEG measures one parameter of brain function in the living patient and can be performed repeatedly so that the course of recovery can be monitored. The EEG, therefore, offers potential usefulness in localizing the site of pathology and following the course of aphasia.

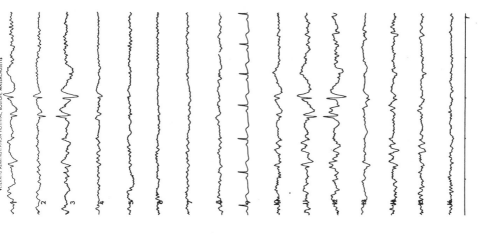

Figure 5-1a and b. *An electroencephalogram showing a clear cut spike focus in the left temporal region. The numbers of the individual channels on 5-1b are indicated on the montage (5-1a). Channel 9 is an EKG monitor.*

Many drawbacks exist in the utilization of the EEG in aphasia, however; the most important one is that the EEG at best offers imprecise anatomical localizing information. A carelessly read EEG can actually implicate the incorrect hemisphere, but even more significant is the fact that the EEG provides only a general indication of the site of pathology. The EEG is most accurate for cortical involvement, but only a small portion of the cortical surface is sampled. Subcortical pathology is also reflected in the EEG, but often over an extensive area, making precise localization difficult. Combinations of cortical and subcortical pathology present immense difficulties for localization, usually allowing only general placements ("central," "temporal"), and even these are subject to mislocalization.

Some of the problems in using the EEG for localization may be corrected. One obvious means is through improved electrode placement in place of the standardized systems used in most laboratories for epilepsy screening. Some EEG localization studies have used a grid, dividing the cortical surface into comparatively limited segments with individual electrodes sampling electrical activity within this grid. Another improvisation utilized successfully in children (Lombroso and Erba, 1970) records the EEG after pentothal injection; the barbiturate produces low voltage fast activity in normal cortex but damaged cortex cannot respond in this way. The accentuated difference in surface frequency helps outline the portions of the cortex which are structurally damaged and can be correlated with aphasic symptoms. In expert hands and with careful attention to special techniques, the EEG can be read closely to provide useful localizing information, but in most laboratories the anatomical localizing information available from routine EEG studies remains imprecise.

CEREBRAL ANGIOGRAPHY

Angiographic evaluation of the cerebral arteries is performed on many patients following cerebral vascular accidents, and so angiograms are available on many individuals under study for aphasia. Routine angiography frequently demonstrates the site of major vessel occlusion, and appropriate timing after onset and careful radiographic techniques may allow demonstration of branch vessel occlusion in many cases (Ring, 1969). Most angiograms are performed during the acute stages, often immediately following the onset of vascular disease. They are permanent records, however, and may be read at leisure, so that correlation with aphasia can wait for weeks or months after the procedure is performed. Several studies (Yarnell, Monroe and Sobel, 1976; Rosenfield and Goree, 1975) have utilized angiographic data for correlating the location of cerebral pathology and the presence of fluent or nonfluent aphasia. Very careful study of angiograms performed at the appropriate stage of recovery may even demonstrate the site of occlusion of the small branches of the middle cerebral artery that often underlie aphasia (Ring and Waddington, 1968).

The angiogram has not proved to be a very useful tool for aphasia localization, however. In the first place, angiography is done at a risk to the patient;

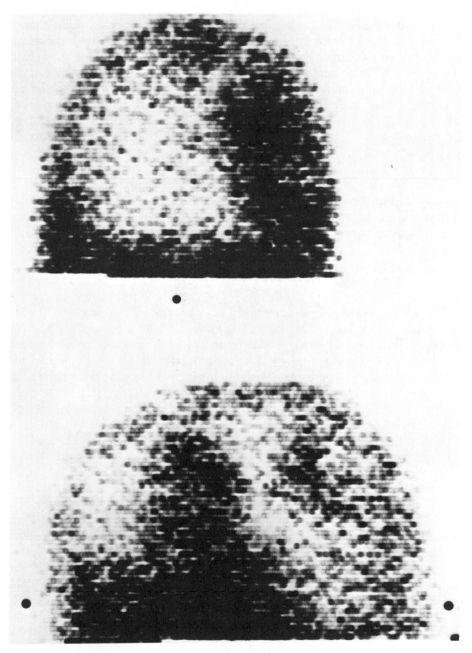

Figure 5-2. *Radioisotope brain scan performed about six weeks after onset of aphasia, outlining a large anterior area of uptake. The upper picture is an AP view, the lower a left lateral scan. The patient originally suffered a global aphasia but evolved into a primarily Broca aphasia picture.*

there is a distinct morbidity (estimates range from 1–4 percent) and there is even a possibility of mortality from the procedure and, therefore, angiography should not be performed without good clinical reason and should never be performed merely to seek aphasia-localizing information. To produce useful cerebral-localizing information, the angiogram must be performed at the correct time, usually a few days after onset of infarction. Even when positive, the angiogram tells only the vessel occluded, not the part of the brain infarcted. Altogether too often the angiogram merely demonstrates a distant occlusion, not the site of infarction. It is perfectly possible for an occluded vessel to have sufficient collateral circulation so that infarction is avoided. Frequently the collateral circulation is not demonstrated and the angiogram can actually be misleading. For these and other reasons, the angiogram has limited usefulness and is rarely used as the sole localization procedure. If available, however, cerebral angiograms deserve review for possible additional localizing information.

RADIOISOTOPE BRAIN SCAN

The advent of the radioisotope brain scan provided the first safe and effective technique for the localization of aphasia-producing lesions in the living patient and stimulated a considerable rebirth of interest in the types of aphasia and the location of the pathology. The procedure is almost totally nonmorbid, comparatively easy to perform, relatively inexpensive and, in good hands, can be read with considerable accuracy. Follow-up studies, utilizing postmortem material, have demonstrated that the isotope brain scan is reasonably accurate in demonstrating both the location of the pathology and the size of the lesion (Howes and Boller, 1978). In the past decade a number of studies have utilized radioisotope brain scan localizations of pathology to correlate with aphasia syndromes (Benson, 1967; Kertesz, Lesk and McCabe, 1977).

The isotope brain scan also has a number of technical drawbacks, however. In vascular cases there is a comparatively short period during which the scan will be positive. This period usually begins about 7–10 days post onset and continues for 6 to 12 weeks post onset (dependent on the size of the lesion). Scans done outside this "window" often fail to show any indication of pathology. Also, most of the commercially available isotope recording equipment currently used performs a rapid scan but produces an image that is small, making the reading of exact neuroanatomical localization almost impossible. The crude apparati originally designed to record isotope uptake produced larger images and allowed better neuroanatomical localization. These procedures had another defect, however; the patient had to remain immobile for a prolonged period while the image was recorded and the scan was often obscured by movement artifact. In addition, most isotope brain scans offer only limited information concerning the depth of the lesion. In sum, the major defect in the use of the radioisotope brain scan has been an inexactness of anatomic localization.

The isotope scan, when positive, does offer accurate information concerning the hemisphere involved, and is usually reliable in demonstrating the lobe of the brain; but it may be unreliable concerning accurate placement of the lesion as to specific gyrus or deep nucleus involved. Despite these limitations, the isotope brain scan has provided valuable localizing information for aphasia correlation and can still be used for this purpose.

REGIONAL CEREBRAL BLOOD FLOW STUDIES

In recent years several independent groups of investigators have developed techniques to demonstrate alterations in cerebral blood flow. Radioactive isotopes are injected (or inhaled) into the carotid artery and simultaneous radioactivity counts are made from a number of areas over the scalp. Comparisons are made between the "counts" from different areas of the brain reflecting the amounts of blood carrying isotopes in the underlying portions of the brain. The technique is technically complex but appears to offer promise for research. Among many studies attempted with this technique has been the demonstration of alterations in blood flow (isotope activity) in specific areas of the brain during performance of language tasks. Thus, reading increases uptake in the more posterior language area, speaking in the more anterior portions and automatic speech (counting, recitation of alphabet, etc.) produces bilaterally-increased uptake (Ingvar and Schwartz, 1974; Larsen, Skinhøj and Lassen, 1978). Following cerebral pathology the patterns of isotope uptake are altered, offering another potentially useful localizing tool (Meyer et al, 1978).

Drawbacks to the cerebral blood flow technique include the fact that it provides only a two-dimensional view, with no information on the depth of the lesion. Invasion of the carotid or femoral artery with a catheter is done at risk to the patient, but for technical reasons it is still the preferred route to introduce isotope. Because of the these limitations the technique has yet to be standardized so there are no recognized patterns for correlation. Regional cerebral blood flow studies are available in only a few laboratories at present and it seems probable that the technique will remain a research tool. As such, however, it may well provide basic information correlating language function and cerebral activity.

Recent technical advances have produced an apparatus utilizing a computerized record of isotope emissions from the brain (emission computerized tomography). While still in the early development stages this technique, which utilizes rapidly degraded isotopes injected intravenously, holds considerable promise for language research. Not only may this unit provide information concerning localization of aphasia-producing pathology, but it may outline cerebral functions (cerebral blood flow, cerebral metabolism) in both normal and abnormal language situations.

COMPUTERIZED TOMOGRAPHY

The relatively new technique of computerized axial tomography (CAT) has already proved useful in aphasia localization and appears destined to become the major diagnostic tool of neurology. The technique is comparatively simple, nonmorbid and is already widely used. CAT scans can be performed multiple times, thus providing follow-up information during recovery. Many types of pathology remain visible permanently, providing useful localizing information in patients who have been aphasic for many years. In fact, some vascular lesions become far more distinct late in the recovery stage and remain clearly outlined over the years. The CAT scan appears superior to any other currently available tool (with the possible exception of the postmortem exam) in demonstrating deep structural pathology, and it successfully demonstrates a wide variety of abnormalities including tumor, hematoma, infarct and trauma.

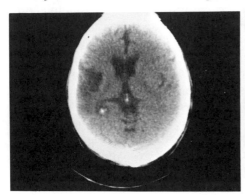 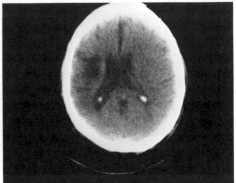

Figure 5-3. Computerized axial tomogram (CAT) demonstrating a moderately old (about 3 months) infarct in the left frontal lobe involving Broca's area but extending to the insula area deep and posterior to the frontal lobe. The patient had severe verbal output disturbance.

With present CAT techniques there are some difficulties, however. Pathology may be indistinct because it has the same density as the surrounding normal tissue. Similarly, the size of a lesion may be exaggerated, particularly if a contrast medium is used to enhance the scan and demonstrates edema surrounding the pathological lesion. The CAT scan, at least as presently used, is not as successful in detailing cortical areas involved by pathology as in outlining damage to subcortical areas. The original scanning devices operated slowly, introducing complicating movement artifact. Newer models have compensated, providing both speedier scanning and better resolution, but at the price of higher radiation dosage. The CAT scan has now developed a small degree of risk. By far the biggest drawback to the use of CAT for cerebral localization is the contemporary technique of angling the tomogram (slice). The angle of the slice is quite unlike any brain slice usually studied, demanding reorientation of anatomical landmarks, and it can lead to many problems in localization. In fact, when the CAT scan is carelessly read or interpreted by a person unsophisticated in neuroanatomy, the localizing information may be not only inaccurate but, worse, completely misleading.

When properly used and interpreted the CAT scan offers immense usefulness for aphasia localization. Excellent results have been obtained from formal studies (Naeser and Hayward, 1978) and the future potential for this tool is immense. Technical improvement, particularly changes in the angle of the tomographic slices, should allow easier and more accurate anatomical localization. Similarly, continued improvements promise better resolution, a very significant factor for accurate anatomical localization. Of all the localizing techniques mentioned in this section, the CAT scan offers the brightest promise for the future. With the widespread use of CAT scanning, the localization of aphasia-producing lesions should become widely practiced, much better understood and generally accepted.

THE LANGUAGE (SPEECH) AREA

On the basis of a variety of localizing techniques many aphasic investigators over the past century have compiled evidence suggesting that one portion of the brain was essential for language. Most frequently this has been called the "speech area;" with the definitions used here, however, the regions discussed actually subserve language and would be better called "the language area."

Most studies outlining the portion of the brain necessary for language have

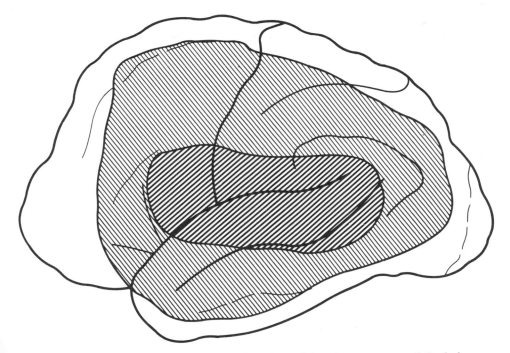

Figure 5-4. *Diagram showing general outline of the "language area." Pathology involving the inner, darker lined area on the left hemisphere almost invariably leads to clinical aphasia whereas pathology in the outer lined area may or may not produce aphasia; involvement of the outermost unshaded area rarely is associated with aphasia.*

been based on war wounds (Marie and Foix, 1917; Head, 1926; Kleist, 1934; Schiller, 1947; Conrad, 1954; Russel and Espir, 1961, Luria, 1970) and illustrate the portion of the brain where overlying injury is most likely to produce aphasia. A second, quite different method was used by Penfield and co-workers (1959) who mapped out areas of the brain significant for language by recording the results of electrical stimulation to the cortex. The results of these studies show general agreement and it appears reasonable to discuss a language area that occupies a sizable portion of the left hemisphere.

As illustrated in Figure 5-4, there is a central, perisylvian area in which damage is very likely to produce aphasia (from 94–97 percent in Luria's series). The central area is surrounded by a larger region, still on the cortical surface, where the percentage of skull trauma cases causing aphasia is smaller but still notable. The remainder of the left cortical surface is only infrequently the site of aphasia-producing lesions; in fact, there is good reason to suspect that, in the few cases of aphasia associated with skull trauma over these more peripheral areas, the actual language involvement stems from distant damage to the language area.

While it appears correct to speak of a language area, roughly as illustrated in Figure 5-4, it must be remembered that none of these studies dealt with the effects of subcortical damage, a situation that is still poorly understood. At best, studies outlining the language area have been uniformly crude. Nonetheless, a left cortical language area appears so consistently from so many localization studies that it seems worthy of acceptance.

6

Classifications of Aphasia

Dating at least from the time of Wernicke, clinicians, particularly neurologists, have demonstrated an almost overwhelming tendency to separate varieties of aphasia on the basis of clusters of language symptoms. The resulting aphasic syndromes represent one of the most confusing aspects of the complex topic of language disturbance. The word *syndrome* and what it represents to different investigators has become a significant part of the confusion. In broad terms, a syndrome can be considered a group of findings, signs and/or symptoms which occur together in a given disease process with sufficient frequency to suggest the presence of that disease process. Although variability, inexactness and incompleteness are commonplace in the constitution of medical syndromes, knowledge of these clusterings has proved immensely helpful to practitioners of medicine. An accomplished clinician once stated that a syndrome was not something concrete, but rather a bit of fantasy invented by the physician to aid in comprehending the intricacies of medical symptomatology (Posner, 1975). As such, syndromes can be considered both imaginary and real. Medical syndromes do not exist as fixed, consistent entities, and as such they may be considered imaginary; however, when the presence of a particular grouping of findings indicates the underlying process with acceptable frequency the syndrome develops a meaning (reality) of its own. Aphasia, as a medical disorder involving the brain, includes a number of different clusters of signs and symptoms and the study of these syndromes has occupied a significant position in the investigation of aphasia.

Unfortunately, many individuals discussing aphasia consider an aphasic syndrome to be a fixed group of language findings and that each finding must invariably be present if a specific disorder is to be diagnosed. An exact syndrome is just as rare in aphasia as in any other medical disorder and many investigators interpret this variability negatively, implying that the syndromes of aphasia have little validity. In one sense this is true; the individual components of the syndrome are not firm and fixed and a specific syndrome is not an invariable result of either a specific process or a specific anatomical localization. In a broader sense, however, there is a strong tendency for the features of aphasia to bunch together into a few comparatively consistent clusters. Hughlings Jackson (1932) correctly observed that the language characteristics of an aphasic patient represented the undamaged residual, the patient's language capability minus those functions made inoperative by brain damage. The resulting cluster of residual language features were recognized early and led to the outlining of multiple syndromes, those of aphasia.

Another widely held but incorrect interpretation of the meaning of a syndrome has led to additional confusion. Many investigators, both clinicians and nonphysicians, expect a reciprocal action; if a given set of findings (syndrome) indicates pathology in a specific anatomic location, then the syndrome should be present whenever pathology involves that area. This is not so, as has been amply proved by innumerable cases showing destruction of a specified portion of the language area (such as Broca's area or the arcuate fasciculus) without aphasia or with unexpected language findings. Not infrequently such findings have been interpreted to mean that the syndrome approach is useless. The definition of a syndrome does not support this interpretation; the syndrome is the collection of symptoms suggesting the location or type of pathology, not the invariable result of pathology involving a given site. This subtle but significant distinction is generally accepted in medicine and is essential for understanding the syndromes of aphasia.

Equally important, no single symptom within a syndrome can be used to indicate the location of neuropathology. This point has been thoroughly defended by Geschwind (1977) who notes that hypotension, scattered dermal pigmentation and low serum sodium do not have specific diagnostic value individually but when they occur together the diagnosis of Addison's disease with pathology in the adrenal glands is probable. Similarly, language-related symptoms such as comprehension disturbance, agraphia, right-left disorientation and many others do not have localizing value individually, but when combined with other findings in a specific grouping they often indicate a specific disorder with specific localization. This is a syndrome.

The syndromology of aphasia became overdeveloped and confusing before the advent of the strong antilocalizationist trend and those who discussed syndromes bore much of the attack of the nonphysicians against the rigid, mechanistic, localizationist viewpoint. Truthfully, however, the rigid, concrete entities most often criticized by these investigators were their own invention, not syndromes in the accepted medical sense. The syndromes of aphasia have survived the onslaughts of the holists and remain a major tool in attempts to understand language disturbances. Idiosyncratic use of aphasia syndromes by various investigators, however, has produced more confusion than clarity, and to understand the place of the aphasic syndromes the many different classifications of the syndromes must be compared.

The short historical background given in Chapter 2 illustrates that many individuals, often in poor communication with one another and just as often in open disagreement, have influenced thinking about aphasia. Many subdivided the varieties of aphasia, emphasizing their personal interests and producing their own syndromes. This led directly to the classifying of subtypes, and as a result aphasia has become one of the most overclassified of all disturbances in neurology, a field in which excessive classifying already abounds. Probably more than any other single aspect, the broad proliferation of different classifications and the consequent confusion has produced the difficulty most students experience with the topic. A single name (e.g. semantic aphasia) may be used in two classifications to represent strikingly different clinical syndromes. The "chaos" outlined by Head (1926) referred directly to the classifications introduced in the first 50 years of aphasia investigation. Antilocalizationists, following Marie, attempted to do without differentiation of symptom clusters but found that they still needed classifications (Marie and Foix, 1917). The confusion has been compounded further by the linguists, speech pathologists and psychologists and other nonphysicians who have introduced classifications featuring their own specialized jargons. In many instances these later classifications contain the same syndromes, disguised by totally different names. A careful study of the classifications is mandatory to the understanding of the aphasia syndromes.

One method of circumventing this problem has been the use of simple dichotomies to classify the aphasias; most contemporary clinicians use one or more of these dichotomies when discussing aphasia. Probably the most widely used is the expressive-receptive division stressed by Weisenburg and McBride (1935). While frequently used, this concept is adequate only as a gross description and is inherently misleading. Even the authors freely admitted that this classification was inadequate and could lead to mistaken interpretation. Almost every patient with aphasia has some degree of expressive abnormality and, similarly, a pure receptive aphasia, one without any hint of expressive problem, is extremely rare. If carefully defined and used accordingly the expressive-receptive dichotomy can be useful, but in inept hands it tends to be misleading.

Another widely used dichotomy is the division into motor and sensory types originally suggested by Wernicke. As most sensory activities are carried out in the posterior portions of the cortex and most motor activities are controlled by the anterior or frontal regions, this dichotomy links language problems with the localization of basic cerebral functions. The division into motor and sensory can thus claim utility but fails to depict the many other features that distinguish the varieties of aphasia. The same can be said for two additional subclassifications of aphasia used frequently in the past decade, the fluent-nonfluent (Benson, 1967) and the anterior-posterior (Goodglass and Kaplan, 1972) dichotomies. Each has a validity and a usefulness but neither adequately characterizes the distinguishing features of most varieties of aphasia.

The most complete nonclassification was suggested by Marie (1906) when he accepted only one type of aphasia, the "sensory" aphasia originally described by Wernicke. In this "classification" all language defect syndromes consist of "aphasia," as defined above, plus involvement of neighborhood motor or sensory functions; the combinations of various neurologic dysfunctions with "aphasia" produce the rich variations of symptomatology seen in the clinic. This holistic view became widely accepted and immensely powerful, reaching its zenith with the work of Schuell (1964) and J. R. Brown (1968) whose writings on aphasia strongly emphasize the "one aphasia" concept.

Brown visualized a "central language process" (CLP) and aphasia was the result of damage to this central process. He also hypothesized a number of "peripheral language processors" (PLP) involved in abstracting (analyzing) sensory input or in programming verbal output. CLP was analogous to an inner speech mechanism whose function was to transform internal meaning into language and language into internal meaning. While Brown considered CLP a

Table 6-1. CLASSIFICATIONS OF APHASIA

Benson 1979	Broca 1865	Bastian 1869	Wernicke (1851) Lichtheim 1885	Pick 1913	Head 1926	Weisenburg & McBride 1933	Kleist 1934
Broca	Aphemia		Cortical motor	Expressive	Verbal	Expressive	Word muteness
Wernicke	Verbal amnesia	Amnesia	Cortical sensory	Impressive	Syntactic	Receptive	Word deafness
Conduction			Conduction				Repetition
Transcortical motor			Transcortical motor				
Transcortical sensory			Transcortical sensory		Nominal		
Mixed transcortical							
Anomic				Amnesic	Semantic	Amnesic	Amnesic
Global			Total	Total		Expressive-receptive	
Alexia with agraphia		Word blindness					
Alexia without agraphia							
Aphemia			Subcortical motor				Anarthric
Pure word deafness		Word deafness	Subcortical sensory				Word sound deafness

Nielsen 1938	Goldstein 1948	Brain 1961	Gloning Gloning/Hoff 1963	Bay 1964	Wepman 1964	Luria 1966	Russell & Espir 1961
Broca	Central motor	Broca	Motor	Cortical dysarthria	Syntactic	Efferent motor	Motor
Wernicke	Wernicke sensory Central	Central Central	Sensory Conduction	Sensory Sensory	Jargon, pragmatic	Sensory Afferent motor	Central Central
Transcort. motor	Transcort. motor			Echolalia		Dynamic	
Transcort. sensory	Transcort. sensory Mixed echolalia					Acoustic amnestic	
Amnesic	Amnesic	Nominal Total or global	Amnestic	Pure	Semantic	Semantic	Alexia
Subcort. motor	Peripheral motor Peripheral sensory	Pure word dumbness Pure word deafness	Pure word deafness				

Table 6-1. CLASSIFICATIONS OF APHASIA (Continued)

Benson & Geschwind 1971	Brown 1972	Adams & Victor 1977	Kertesz & Phipps 1977	Hecaen & Albert 1978
Broca	Broca	Broca	Broca	Pure motor
Wernicke	Wernicke	Wernicke	Wernicke	Sensory
Conduction	Conduction	Conduction	Efferent & Afferent cond.	Conduction
Transcortical motor			Transcortical motor	Transcort. motor
Transcortical sensory	Semantic		Transcortical sensory	Transcort. sensory
Isolation of speech area		Isolation of speech area	Isolation	
Anomic	Anomia	Anomic	Anomic	Amnesic
Global		Total	Global	
Alexia with agraphia				Alexia with agraphia
Alexia without agraphia		Pure word blindness		Pure alexia
Aphemia		Pure word muteness		
Pure word deafness	Pure word deafness	Pure word deafness		Pure word deafness

single, separate and unitary language mechanism, Maruszewski (1975) has pointed out that even in this model, language processing is indeed a multifactorial phenomenon.

The linguist Jakobson strongly refuted the holistic approach (1964) and subsequent neuropsychological studies tend to support a diverse organizational system for language. The "chaos" of the reductionistic classifications cannot be simply discarded and, therefore, must be analyzed further. Fortunately, beneath all the philosophic and semantic babble concerning nomenclature, a core of reasonableness can be discovered. As Howes noted (1964), discussion of aphasia with individuals experienced in the field reveals considerable agreement on most salient points. In many ways it would appear that the academic and technical descriptions of the aphasic disturbances act as roadblocks, not aids, to understanding. Indeed, if one can see through the smoke screen of the intellectually derived confusion, the same few basic clinical syndromes appear in most classifications, albeit under different names. The number of such entities is finite and the types of aphasia presented in one classification can almost always be correlated with the types of aphasia in another classification.

To aid the study of the many classifications, a table has been constructed which lists (and allows correlation) of a number of the historically more important classifications of aphasia.

A cursory glance at Table 6-1 reveals an apparently overwhelming confusion, both in the types of aphasia and in the terminology suggested. Nonetheless, correlations between some of the entities of the various classifications are obvious. While often based on separate and even antagonistic theories, the clusters of clinical findings used in the various classifications possess a consis-

Table 6-2. SYNDROMES OF APHASIA

Perisylvian Aphasia Syndromes	Nonlocalizing aphasic syndromes
Broca aphasia	Anomic aphasia
Wernicke aphasia	Global aphasia
Conduction aphasia	Alexia
Borderzone Aphasia Syndromes	Parietal-temporal alexia
Transcortical motor aphasia	Occipital alexia
Aphasia of anterior cerebral artery	Frontal alexia
infarction	Agraphia
Transcortical sensory aphasia	Related Syndromes
Mixed transcortical aphasia	Aphemia
Subcortical Aphasia Syndromes	Pure word deafness
The aphasia of Marie's quadrilateral	Apraxia of speech
space	Nonaphasic misnaming
Thalamic aphasia	
Striatal aphasia	
Aphasia from white matter lesions	

tency. For each variety of aphasia listed in Table 6-1, either the clinical features (syndrome), or the location of the pathology or both, have been sufficiently well-described by the author to allow correlation with entities from the other classifications featuring similar constellations of symptoms of pathological locus; syndromes such as those called Broca (motor) aphasia and Wernicke (sensory) aphasia occur in most of the classifications and several other varieties (anomic, conduction) appear in many. A number of additional syndromes may be proposed, however. Table 6-2 lists the syndromes that will be described in this volume.

Most of the syndromes in Table 6-2 can be correlated with syndromes from the other classifications listed in Table 6-1, an exercise demonstrating that much of the confusion in the classification of aphasia is artificial. There is far better agreement on the characterizing features of the various syndromes than on the names given to them. Official agreement on nomenclature is not only indicated but appears essential for improved understanding of aphasia. In no way, however, should it be construed that the classification presented in Table 6-2 is necessarily superior to the other classifications. In fact, Table 6-1 rather clearly demonstrates that each classification is attempting to describe, within the confines of the investigator's personal approach to language or language disturbance, the same entities. It is the terminology, not the syndromes, that is so strikingly different and is the source of most of the confusion.

7

Perisylvian Aphasic Syndromes

The first three syndromes noted in Table 6-2 have two notable similarities. Each of the syndromes features a serious difficulty in repetition of spoken language as a prominent clinical finding and, anatomically, the sites of pathology consistently described in these disorders are located about the sylvian fissure of the dominant hemisphere. The three disorders to be discussed in this chapter are among the best known and most widely accepted of all aphasic syndromes. The basic findings of each syndrome will be outlined and then some of the many variations will be presented along with general prognosis and, finally, anatomical correlations.

BROCA APHASIA

Paul Broca was the first to describe an aphasic syndrome and correlate it with underlying pathology (1861a, 1861b, 1865). For over a century a variety of aphasia bearing his name has evolved and a specified anatomic localization for this disturbance has been widely accepted. As documented in Table 6-1, the same syndrome has been given many other names; for instance, the same findings have been called motor aphasia, efferent motor aphasia, expressive aphasia, anterior aphasia, verbal aphasia, etc., and it has even been denied, emphatically, that this particular group of findings indicates the presence of aphasia (Marie, 1906a, b, c). Despite all of this, the term Broca aphasia is almost universally recognized and appears to be the least objectionable for this syndrome.

The basic syndrome of Broca aphasia can be outlined by description of the six major language functions presented in Table 7-1. There are many variations of these symptoms, however, that deserve careful attention.

The verbal output in Broca aphasia can be described quite accurately as nonfluent (review Ch. 4 for detailed descriptions of nonfluent verbal output). It is sparse, poorly articulated, consists of very short phrases (characteristically one word in length or, following improvement, telegraphic), is produced with considerable effort, particularly on initiation of speech and is strikingly dysprosodic. The output consists almost exclusively of substantives such as nouns, action verbs, significant modifiers or stock phrases (cliches). The marked deficiency or absence of syntactical, structural words (functors) makes the output strikingly abnormal, even to casual observation. The comparatively

Table 7-1. BASIC LANGUAGE CHARACTERISTICS
OF BROCA APHASIA

Conversational speech	Nonfluent
Comprehension of spoken language	Relatively normal
Repetition of spoken language	Abnormal
Confrontation-Naming	Abnormal
Reading: Aloud	Abnormal
Comprehension	Normal or abnormal
Writing	Abnormal

rich substantive quality of the output, however, enables the patient with Broca aphasia to communicate some ideas despite severe deficiencies in verbal output. For some, the output is limited to repetitive output of a single word or expression, a *verbal stereotypy*. At times the stereotypy can be inflected allowing some sense of meaning to be communicated through the single verbalization. The defect in articulation has been called by many terms (phonemic disintegration, cortical dysarthria, verbal apraxia, etc.) and, while common, may not be considered present in an individual case of Broca aphasia. In fact, almost any of the above features can be missing in individuals who would still be considered to have Broca aphasia. While the fully developed syndrome includes the verbal output features noted above, variations which omit one or several output features are so common as to be the rule rather than the exception.

Comprehension of spoken language in Broca aphasia is always qualitatively better than verbal output, but again considerable variation, from near normal to distinctly abnormal, is seen regularly. Some authorities insist that any abnormality of comprehension excludes a diagnosis of Broca aphasia but this demand for purity has never been widely accepted. Most patients with Broca aphasia have some degree of comprehension defect and there are several distinctive characteristics of this comprehension deficit which appear useful diagnostically. One frequent defect is an inability to handle multiple bits of information in sequence. A patient with Broca aphasia may readily identify individual items or body parts named by the examiner but when asked to point to multiple items or body parts in a specific sequence may fail at a level of only two or three items. Whether this represents a disturbance of the ability to perform a sequential motor act or a defective auditory span is unsettled. Whatever the underlying explanation, an inability to point sequentially is a common comprehension defect in Broca aphasia. Of a somewhat similar but not necessarily related nature, many patients with Broca aphasia have difficulty understanding relational words (bigger-smaller, up-down, within-without) and recent reports (Zurif, Carramazza and Myerson, 1972) suggest that problems in the comprehension of most grammatical or syntactical language structures are present in patients with Broca aphasia. The disturbance apparently involves abnormal comprehension of the same terms that Broca aphasia patients omit from their verbal expressions. Despite these difficulties the patient with Broca aphasia can comprehend much of what is said and there is little doubt that the comprehension of spoken language is considerably more intact than the ability to express in language.

Repetition of spoken language is always abnormal in Broca aphasia; in fact, this finding is a requirement to make this diagnosis. Without a significant abnormality of repetition, a patient with the nonfluent verbal output and comprehension just described would have transcortical motor aphasia (see Ch. 8). Despite the obvious abnormality of repetition in Broca aphasia, however, this function is often superior to the spontaneous verbal output and is frequently misinterpreted as normal repetition. Careful evaluation will show this is not so. One striking difficulty of repetition commonly noted in Broca aphasia is the selective inability to repeat the same syntactic, grammatical, linguistic structures omitted from spontaneous output. Thus, when a patient with Broca aphasia is asked to say "the big black dog" he may produce "black, dog," with considerable coaching add the "big," but consistently fail to repeat "the." This becomes more pronounced if the patient is asked to repeat sentences with substantive words plus modifiers ("the boy and the girl are at home"), often performed merely by repetition of the substantive words ("boy-girl-home").

Series speech should always be tested in cases of suspected Broca aphasia. The patient often performs considerably better in automatic activities such as counting, or naming the days of the week or the months; even the articulation often improves greatly with these automatic verbal tasks. It is striking to note how well a patient articulates when reciting a series but cannot articulate the same words correctly in a repetition task. Singing familiar melodies often improves the verbal output in patients with Broca aphasia; there is little or no carryover of the improved pronunciation of singing or automatic speech into spontaneous verbal output, however.

Confrontation-naming is invariably poor in individuals with the Broca aphasia syndrome but, just as with repetition, may appear relatively preserved when compared to the extreme paucity of names in conversational output. Serious problems of articulation are frequently noted during tests of naming. Broca aphasia patients often accept cues (prompting) well, appearing to benefit from them in overcoming problems in pronunciation or initiating articulation. The Broca aphasic who fails to name an object on presentation may name it readily when the initial syllable is pronounced or even when the lip movement necessary for the initial syllable is demonstrated by the examiner. Similarly, an open-ended sentence in which the desired name is the final word ("you pound a nail with a ____") is often successful in aiding the patient to produce the name of an object (Barton, Maruszewski and Urrea, 1969). While this trait may occur in other types of aphasia, accepting cues is most characteristic of the Broca type of aphasia.

As could be expected, most patients with Broca aphasia have great difficulty (almost total failure) when attempting to read out loud. Somewhat unexpected, most of these patients also have some degree of difficulty comprehending written material (see Ch. 11 for additional description of the reading problems of anterior aphasia). While many patients with Broca aphasia understand some written material, they find reading extremely difficult and avoid doing it (Benson, 1977). There are occasional exceptions, however: some patients with all the other language characteristics of Broca aphasia do read well.

Writing is abnormal in Broca aphasia. Characteristically, the handwriting consists of oversized, poorly formed letters, multiple misspellings and the omission of letters. Most patients with Broca aphasia have right hemiplegia necessitating the use of the left hand for writing. The written output is notably inferior, however, to that produced by normal individuals writing with their nondominant hand. The writing defect affects the ability to write both on command and to dictation and there is even abnormality in the patient's ability to copy written material (see Ch. 12 for additional descriptions of aphasic agraphia).

The routine neurologic examination in cases of Broca aphasia almost invariably provides diagnostically useful findings but there can be considerable variation in these findings. Most frequently (over 80 percent of cases), some degree of right-sided motor weakness, often a full right hemiplegia or significant hemiparesis, will be present (Howes and Geschwind, 1964). If the defect is incomplete the paresis is usually maximal in the upper extremity with a lesser involvement in the lower extremity. Hyperactive reflexes and abnormal pathological reflexes are frequently present on the involved side. Ideomotor apraxia, an inability to carry out, on command, a task that can be done spontaneously (Geschwind, 1967a) frequently involves the "nonpathological" left hand of patients with Broca aphasia. With this difficulty, a person with a right hemiplegia, when asked to make a fist, salute or some other manual task with the left hand, may produce only clumsy approximate movements; if asked to demonstrate use of a comb or a toothbrush, the same patient may replace a body part (fingers) for parts of the pretended object.

Sensory abnormality is not consistent but occurs with fair frequency in Broca aphasia. The sensory loss may be severe, including loss of both pain and cortical sensory functions, suggesting a deep extension to involve medullary structures. In other individuals with Broca aphasia the sensory loss is much milder or even entirely absent. If a severe hemisensory defect is present at the onset but clears rapidly, a unilateral inattention syndrome is suggested (Kennard, 1939; Heilman, 1979) rather than a true sensory loss. Similarly, the visual sensory findings vary tremendously in cases of Broca aphasia. Not infrequently a conjugate deviation to the left or a significant degree of gaze paresis will be present at onset but disappears within a few days or weeks, again suggesting unilateral inattention (see Ch. 16 for additional discussion of this fascinating complication). Neglect of the right side may persist, however, possibly producing some language comprehension difficulty, particularly in reading. Persistent visual field defects do occur with Broca aphasia, but not as commonly as in other varieties of aphasia; many neurologists suggest that a persistent visual field defect indicates more posterior neuroanatomical involvement.

Localization of the site of pathology in cases of Broca aphasia has been the subject of many studies, beginning with the original presentations of Broca (1861a, 1861b) utilizing clinical-neuropathological correlations. Many studies of

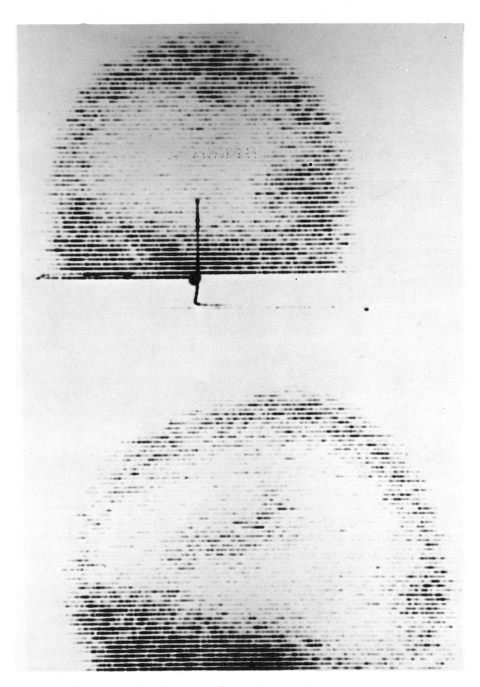

Figure 7-1. *Isotope brain scan (AP and left lateral) showing a comparatively small area of increased uptake sharply localized to the left posterior-inferior frontal area with moderately deep extension. Clinically the patient showed the characteristics of Broca aphasia.*

the aphasic disturbances produced by war-induced brain injury have localized Broca (motor) aphasia to the dominant posterior-inferior frontal lobe (Schiller, 1947; Russell and Espir, 1961; Luria, 1970). The radioisotope brain scan (Kertesz, Lesk and McCabe, 1977) and the CT scan (Naeser and Hayward, 1978) have all placed the pathology in cases of Broca aphasia in this same general area. Figure 7-1 shows the increased radioactive uptake in a case of Broca aphasia, clearly demonstrating the location of pathology in the posterior frontal area. Figure 7-2 shows a CAT scan from another Broca aphasic; note the extensive depth of the pathology, a factor not apparent in the isotope scan. Both procedures offer valuable localizing information and these improved techniques for locating pathology within the brains of living subjects supports the classic localization.

There has been considerable discussion about the course of recovery in Broca aphasia in recent years (Mohr, 1973). Two general patterns have been suggested. One is a severe aphasic disturbance, often considered global at the beginning, that over a period of days, weeks or months evolves into the classic picture of Broca aphasia noted above. A second course begins with mutism and can evolve into either aphemia (see Ch. 13) or Broca aphasia. The latter course generally has a better prognosis for eventual recovery than the one starting with global aphasia. It would appear that if a patient shows the characteristics of Broca aphasia at the onset, the prognosis for recovery is comparatively good, often rapidly improving to a level of minimal language disturbance.

Various types of pathology can produce Broca aphasia including trauma, tumor, infection, abscess and others. By far the most common cause is cerebral vascular disease. Occlusion of one or several tributaries of the middle cerebral artery feeding the inferior frontal region is the most common cause of Broca aphasia except in wartime military practice.

Despite almost incessant disagreement over the exact boundaries of the neuroanatomical site involved in Broca aphasia, there is general agreement on the central importance of the posterior-interior portion of the dominant frontal lobe, particularly the pars triangularis and opercularis (also known as F3, Brodmann's area 44 or simply Broca's area). It has been suggested (Henschen, 1922; Kleist, 1934a) that fully developed Broca aphasia demands deep subcortical pathology as well as damage to the frontal cortex. With the advent of modern diagnostic techniques this statement has been amply confirmed (Mohr et al, 1978). In fact, it can be considered that some of the variation in symptomatology in cases of Broca aphasia may depend on the various sites of the deep pathology and there can be little doubt that the symptoms of the syndrome vary with the size of the lesion (Mohr, 1973). The larger the lesion, the more widespread the effect. A second, less obvious but apparently real explanation for the variations in the syndrome concerns the stage of the disorder. The clinical picture does improve and examinations performed soon after onset show more complex problems than do later examinations. A third explanation, also obvious but not widely accepted at present, concerns the exact neuroanatomic sites involved by pathology. While the frontal operculum defect is generally recognized, defects in many other areas such as the callosal path-

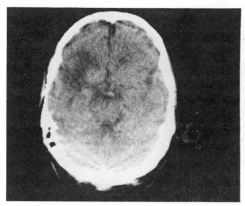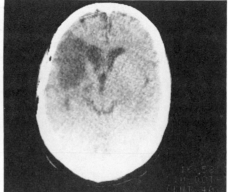

Figure 7-2. CAT scan showing a large area of infarction in the left posterior frontal area. Note the extensive involvement deep to Broca's area. The patient had a severe Broca aphasia.

ways connecting to the right hemisphere, cortical-cortical connections with the posterior language areas, motor pathways passing to the brain stem motor articulation areas and/or involvement of neighboring frontal lobe cortical areas, anterior or superior to the operculum, all probably affect the language picture. In addition, there may be individual variation among patients concerning the involvement of an anatomical site with a specific language function. While the many variables produce an almost automatic basis for disagreement, there is almost universal recognition of the syndrome picture we have called Broca aphasia and general acceptance that this syndrome indicates pathology involving the frontal operculum and cerebral tissues deep to this area.

WERNICKE APHASIA

Wernicke aphasia is also widely recognized, although not so fully accepted as a name for a specific aphasia syndrome. Essentially identical aphasia syndromes have been called sensory aphasia, receptive aphasia, central aphasia and many other names. Nonetheless, most individuals dealing with aphasia recognize Wernicke aphasia as a specific syndrome and the term will be retained for this distinct cluster of findings. No matter what name is recognized, this syndrome is widely accepted as a true aphasic condition. Table 7-2 lists the major language findings in Wernicke aphasia.

The verbal output in Wernicke aphasia is characterized by the features of fluency (see Ch. 4) with a normal or even excessive number of words produced per minute. In fact, the greatest quantity of words produced by aphasics come from those with Wernicke aphasia. These patients often augment, by adding additional syllables to the ends of words or additional words or phrases to the end of sentences. The output can become so excessive that the patient speaks continually unless forcefully stopped by the examiner, a phenomenon called

Table 7-2. BASIC LANGUAGE CHARACTERISTICS
OF WERNICKE APHASIA

Conversational speech	Fluent, paraphasic
Comprehension of spoken language	Abnormal
Repetition of spoken language	Abnormal
Confrontation-Naming	Abnormal
Reading: Aloud	Abnormal
Comprehension	Abnormal
Writing	Abnormal

press of speech or *logorrhea,* an aphasic output almost diagnostic for Wernicke aphasia. There is little or no effort needed to produce the verbal output, the phrase length is normal (5–8 words) and in most cases there is an acceptable grammatical structure and no problems of either articulation or prosody. The content of the verbal output in Wernicke aphasia almost invariably shows a deficiency of meaningful, substantive words, so that despite the many words produced the ideas of the individual are not effectively conveyed, a phenomenon that can be called *empty speech.*

Another phenomenon frequently noted in Wernicke aphasia is paraphasia. The most characteristic type of substitution is verbal (semantic), the substitution of one recognizable word for another, but mixtures with literal paraphasias and neologisms are not uncommon. If the patient produces an excessive number of words with multiple paraphasic substitutions including all three types, the output becomes completely incomprehensible, a gibberish that has been termed *jargon aphasia.*

Jargon is not confined to cases of Wernicke aphasia. In a study of neologistic jargon, a verbal output featuring various types of paraphasia but with an excess of neologisms, Kertesz and Benson (1970) demonstrated that recovery occasioned one of two separate syndromes, either a prevalence of semantic paraphasia and other findings suggesting Wernicke aphasia or a prevalence of phonemic substitutions (literal paraphasia) and a diagnosis of conduction aphasia. Jargon aphasia should be reserved as a descriptive term and not used to signify a full language syndrome.

If one can get the patient with Wernicke aphasia started in the proper set, it is often possible to demonstrate comparatively good retention of series speech. Thus tasks like counting, naming the days of the week or the recitation of poems or nursery rhymes may be performed comparatively well.

Along with the fluent, disordered output, a second significant characteristic of Wernicke aphasia is a serious problem in the comprehension of spoken language. When severe, the patient understands absolutely no spoken language; more often it is partial with some ability to understand single words, phrases or even short sentences. Not infrequently, patients with Wernicke aphasia will understand several words when first tested, then fail to comprehend additional words, and if the words originally understood are immediately retested, they will fail to understand these words also. This striking phenomenon, almost pathognomonic of Wernicke aphasia, has been called "fatigue" or "jamming" to suggest the apparent source of difficulty but the true cause of this phenomenon remains unknown. Some patients with Wernicke aphasia show an inability to discriminate separate phonemes (phonemic perception) (Luria, 1966). Thus the ability to discriminate sounds which vary only slightly (ba-pa-da) may be deficient. This has not been true of all patients with the clinical findings of Wernicke aphasia, however.

A striking problem for many patients with Wernicke aphasia is difficulty in changing from one task to another (changing set). If a line of communication is established so that the patient tries to comprehend room object names and the task is then changed (e.g. body parts), total failure of response often results. Many patients with Wernicke aphasia fail in some comprehension tasks but do better in others. The specific tasks succeeded or failed vary considerably among patients with one striking exception. Most patients with Wernicke aphasia, even if severe, successfully carry out whole body commands. Thus many patients who cannot follow any command, nor in any other way demonstrate that they comprehend spoken language, can carry out commands involving the entire body; for instance such complex tasks as holding a bat like a baseball player, doing a waltz step, etc. have been performed on command by patients who have otherwise failed all comprehension tasks. Retention of whole body commands is not universal in Wernicke aphasia, but it is sufficiently common to warrant attention. Many patients with Wernicke aphasia will fail to carry out a commanded limb or bucco-facial activity, but imitation of the activity will be performed well. This observation is not restricted to Wernicke aphasia but is more characteristic of this syndrome than any other.

Repetition of spoken language is invariably disturbed in Wernicke aphasia, usually in a degree related to the disturbance of comprehension. Thus a patient who understands little or nothing will repeat little or nothing, but if an occasional word or phrase is understood, repetition will be successful to the same degree.

Patients with Wernicke aphasia most often either fail totally or produce grossly paraphasic responses when asked to name objects, body parts, etc. on visual confrontation. There are exceptions, however. Some patients with the other findings of the Wernicke aphasia syndrome can produce names upon confrontation far better than expected and disturbed word-finding cannot be considered an essential feature of the syndrome. Nonetheless, serious difficulty in naming is common. It is striking that the names produced by Wernicke aphasics are often contaminated by literal paraphasia. Thus a patient who is producing a copious output liberally laced with verbal paraphasia, when asked to name an object, often produces a neologistic or literal paraphasic facsimile of the desired word. Again this phenomenon is not constant, but the alteration of types of paraphasia between spontaneous output and naming tasks is frequently noted.

Reading is always disturbed, and the degree often parallels the disturbance in spoken language comprehension. The equality of the disturbance is less exact than with repetition, however. Many examiners have remarked on the variations in the comprehension defect between spoken and written language in Wernicke aphasia. In particular, Hecaen (1969) and Hier and Mohr (1978) have demonstrated a bipolar tendency in the comprehension defect of Wernicke aphasia. Some patients show their most striking disturbance in the comprehension of spoken words (word deafness) while others have more difficulty comprehending written words (word blindness). For a diagnosis of Wernicke aphasia there must be considerable disability in comprehending spoken language but also some disturbance in comprehending written language. If reading comprehension is normal, the syndrome is more properly termed "pure word deafness" (see Ch. 13).

The question as to why reading comprehension is disturbed in a disorder featuring an abnormality of auditory language comprehension has been raised frequently. Wernicke offered an explanation that, while still unproved, remains acceptable. He noted that during normal development the child acquires a comparatively complete auditory language before even attempting to learn a visual language. Visual language is then learned through association with the already well-established auditory language. Brain damage that involves the auditory language function can interfere with the visual-verbal association underlying reading, producing an alexia. Another frequently suggested explanation is the entirely mechanical neuroanatomical one suggested by the proximity of Wernicke's area in the temporal lobe and the angular gyrus of the parietal lobe. That the reading disturbance of Wernicke aphasia is identical to the alexia of parietal-temporal pathology and is the result of pathological involvement of this area (see Ch. 11) is difficult to disprove but there is at least some evidence suggesting that purely temporal pathology can produce alexia (Nielsen, 1939). Whatever explanation is correct, all cases of Wernicke aphasia do show difficulty in the comprehension of written language material.

Writing is also abnormal in Wernicke aphasia but the written output is strikingly different from the agraphia of Broca aphasia. The patient with Wernicke aphasia can use his dominant hand for writing and the output consists of well-formed, legible letters combined in the appearance of words; the letters are often combined in a meaningless manner, however. Correctly-produced words may be scattered among the unintelligible combinations (see Ch. 12 for more details of posterior agraphia). In some instances the written output closely resembles the paraphasic spoken output; if the written material were sounded out it would be like the verbal output the patient is presenting as he writes.

The routine neurologic examination is often totally negative in Wernicke aphasia. There is little or no paresis (although a history of a transient paresis, lasting up to a few days at the onset of the disorder, is common). Some degree of cortical sensory disturbance may be present but even this is the exception, not the rule. There are no extraocular motor problems in uncomplicated Wernicke aphasia but a superior quandrantanopsia, suggesting involvement of the temporal radiation of the geniculo-calcarine tract (Meyer's loop), is present with moderate frequency. The visual field defect is the only basic neurologic deficit present in many cases of Wernicke aphasia. The lack of obvious neurologic abnormality easily leads to incorrect diagnosis. In particular, older patients with the striking language disturbance of Wernicke aphasia without notable basic neurologic deficit are mistakenly considered demented, while younger patients are called psychotic and not infrequently treated as schizophrenic. Careful language-testing, particularly good comprehension testing, readily differentiates these states but many patients with Wernicke aphasia are misdiagnosed each year.

Localization of the site of pathology in cases of Wernicke aphasia has been accomplished frequently and by many methods. Wernicke published one case with localization demonstrated by autopsy findings in his original paper (1874); many other autopsy localizations have been reported and other methods (surgical intervention, radioisotope scan, CAT scan) have successfully confirmed the site. Figure 7-3 illustrates a CAT scan from a patient with the clinical findings of Wernicke aphasia.

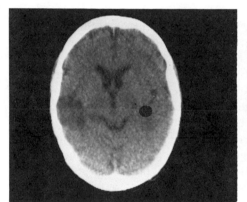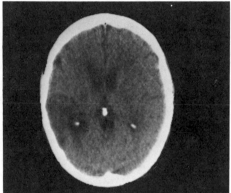

Figure 7-3. *CAT scan showing a moderate sized infarction centered in the left posterior temporal area with extension posteriorly to involve inferior parietal tissues. The patient had the features of Wernicke aphasia.*

There is considerable variation in the course of this disorder. In the first place the classic form of Wernicke aphasia appears to occur in older patients than those with classic Broca aphasia (Obler, Albert, Goodglass, and Benson, 1978). Also, there is less tendency for a favorable outcome. Often the disorder begins with a totally neologistic output, severe comprehension disturbance and an apparent unawareness of the deficit. Serious behavior problems that demand specialized management are frequent (see Ch. 17). With improvement, some ability to recognize spoken words appears. At this stage the slow presentation of auditory material permits far better comprehension than normal or rapid speeds of presentation (Albert and Bear, 1974). With continued improvement, the patient becomes increasingly aware of the problem and concentrates on understanding those around him. Verbal (semantic) paraphasia may continue but decreases in frequency. There can also be an ongoing improvement in reading but this may be entirely absent.

One of the more striking findings of the general examination concerns behavior. Characteristically patients with Wernicke aphasia are unaware of their deficit and, in addition, show a remarkable unconcern. Many begin to suspect that individuals in their environment are the source of their problem. They can become bitterly paranoid, accusing the staff, their family and acquaintances of not listening carefully to what they are saying or not speaking carefully enough to be understood. Paranoid patients can become agitated and can then be dangerous to themselves and others (see Ch. 16). Many patients with Wernicke aphasia can be considered psychotic as they are out of contact with their environment, at least in a verbal sense. Most are not, however, out of contact in a social sense (and, therefore, not truly psychotic), and continued interrelation through gesture and other forms of nonverbal communication can prove very helpful. While the paranoia is the most dramatic, the unawareness and unconcern are far more common behavior problems and often prove diagnostically meaningful.

A variety of pathological entities are known to produce Wernicke aphasia. No only can the disorder be seen after a typical cerebral vascular accident, embolic or thrombotic, but it frequently follows intracerebral hemorrhage involving the temporal lobe. Trauma or tumor are likely to be the cause of the latter. Tumor in the temporal lobe, even without hemorrhage, can produce a picture of Wernicke aphasia, and before the introduction and widespread use of antibiotics, abscess formation in the dominant temporal lobe was a common cause of Wernicke aphasia.

Classically, Wernicke aphasia indicates involvement of the posterior part of the superior temporal gyrus, an area generally considered to be the auditory association cortex and often called Wernicke's area. This area is situated adjacent to the primary auditory cortex (Heschl's gyrus) which may or may not be involved in Wernicke aphasia. Figure 7-4 diagrammatically illustrates Wernicke's area. Considerable variation exists in the symptom picture of Wernicke aphasia, at least partially based on the exact location and extent of the pathology involving the temporal lobe. As always, pathology in this area does not necessarily mean that the syndrome will be present, and there are many reports in the literature documenting negative correlations. The opposite, however, can be stated with considerable confidence: cases featuring the symptom picture of Wernicke aphasia almost invariably have pathology that involves the auditory association area of the dominant hemisphere. The depth of the lesion is another important variable in Wernicke aphasia. Not infrequently the lesion involves Heschl's gyrus or the white matter pathways connecting this region to subcortical sensory centers, producing an added element of receptive disturbance (see pure word deafness in Ch. 13 and the discussion of the varieties of comprehension disturbance in Ch. 15). Posterior or inferior extension of the lesion can probably be linked to increased word blindness and anomia. In practice, most cases that can be labeled Wernicke aphasia tend to have structural damage involving a considerably greater territory than just Wernicke's area.

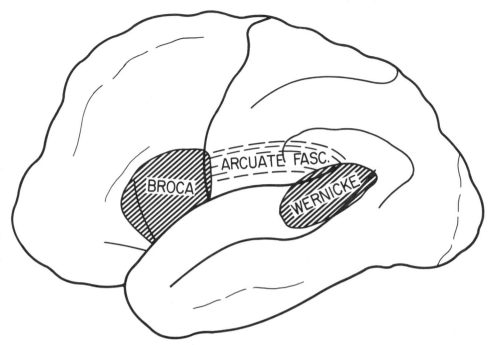

Figure 7-4. *Diagrammatic view of left lateral hemisphere outlining cortical areas commonly associated with Broca and Wernicke aphasia plus a schematic illustration of the arcuate fasciculus, site of pathology in some cases of conduction aphasia.*

CONDUCTION APHASIA

In his 1874 monograph, Wernicke proposed the two types of aphasia and the separate anatomical areas noted above, one in the temporal lobe and the other in the posterior-inferior frontal lobe. He conjectured that an anatomical connection between these areas was necessary and further conjectured that damage to this pathway when neither of the other two language areas were damaged would cause a clinically distinct syndrome. He suggested the term *Leitungsaphasie* for this disorder; this is now called *conduction aphasia.* A variety of aphasia with the characteristics postulated by Wernicke has been demonstrated many times. However, despite excellent clinical descriptions in the literature, complete with pathological findings (Lichtheim, 1885; Kleist, 1934b; Benson et al, 1973), conduction aphasia has not been widely accepted as a separate aphasia entity. Many of the classifications of aphasia outlined in Chapter 6 omit conduction aphasia entirely. Some contemporary investigators believe that conduction aphasia exists only rarely (Luria, 1966) while many others include it with one or another variety of posterior aphasia under a number of more general terms (Russell and Espir, 1961; Brain, 1961). Good language examinations readily separate conduction aphasia from the other varieties, and in our experience conduction aphasia is a specific language disorder syndrome that is seen frequently in the clinic. In two separate studies, conduction aphasia was present in between 10 and 15 percent of aphasic admissions (Benson et al, 1973; Hecaen and Albert, 1978).

Table 7-3. BASIC LANGUAGE CHARACTERISTICS
OF CONDUCTION APHASIA

Conversational speech	Fluent, paraphasic
Comprehension of spoken language	Good to normal
Repetition of spoken language	Abnormal
Confrontation-Naming	Usually abnormal
Reading: Aloud	Abnormal
Comprehension	Good to normal
Writing	Abnormal

The conversational output in conduction aphasia is fluent and paraphasic but the amount of output is notably less than in Wernicke aphasia. The patient not only produces less speech but there are more pauses, usually hesitations for word-finding or difficulty in producing words because of excessive phonemic error. Characteristically the output of conduction aphasia has a broken, dysprosodic quality. It is not infrequent to find that classic examples of conduction aphasia have been called "expressive aphasia" because of the broken output. Several features, however, easily differentiate this output from that of Broca aphasia. Many different four- and five-word phrases are easily and correctly produced. They may be cliches (e.g. "I don't know if I can," "what did you say?") but the phrases are too variable to be classed as stereotypes and have a normal melodic line. The large amount of literal paraphasia in the output is another distinguishing feature. While Broca aphasia may contain some output features that can be classed as literal paraphasia, it is not in the quantity present in conduction aphasia and always occurs in the context of severe dysarthria. In contrast, articulation is excellent in conduction aphasia, even to the point of good pronunciation of the wrong phoneme.

The patient with conduction aphasia often performs adequately in series speech if given a start. Similarly, he or she usually produces words better in singing than in conversational output.

Comprehension of spoken language is strikingly good in conduction aphasia. In some individuals comprehension appears fully normal and in others the difficulty appears limited in the understanding of complex grammatical structures or statements containing multiple key words or phrases. In general, the comprehension of patients with conduction aphasia is fully adequate for normal conversation. In fact, a significant degree of comprehension disturbance makes the diagnosis of conduction aphasia questionable.

In contrast to the normal comprehension, patients with conduction aphasia have serious problems in repeating spoken language. The dramatic difference between repetition and comprehension is an essential feature of this syndrome and is often considered the key finding. Repetition is characteristically contaminated by multiple literal paraphasias, but if asked to repeat numbers or color names, the patient may produce verbal paraphasic substitutions (i.e. an incorrect number). Repetition is strikingly poorer than the ability to produce words in conversational speech. When unable to correctly repeat a word or a phrase, the patient with conduction aphasia often produces an excellent paraphrase (as an example, when asked to say the word "rifle" a soldier said "riffle-ridil, oh hell, I mean gun"). It has been stated that the patient with conduction aphasia has most difficulty repeating grammatical words and that numbers are the easiest to repeat. This is not consistently demonstrated, however. It has also been suggested that the entire repetition problem in conduction aphasia is a defect of auditory span (Warrington and Shallice, 1969) a point of serious disagreement (Tzortzis and Albert, 1974; Strub and Gardner, 1974). There is little disagreement, however, that difficulty in the repetition of spoken language is a key feature of conduction aphasia.

Most patients with conduction aphasia have difficulty in confrontation-naming (Green and Howes, 1977). In some instances the anomia appears to consist entirely of paraphasic substitutions, but a true inability to find a word occurs frequently in conduction aphasia.

Tests of reading ability are striking in many cases of conduction aphasia. Characteristically there is a serious problem in reading out loud with rapid breakdown into severely paraphasic output. In contrast, these same individuals can read silently (for comprehension) with comparative ease. Many instances have been recorded of patients with conduction aphasia who are unable to read a three- or four-word newspaper headline out loud but regularly read the entire newspaper, novels and even textbooks of medicine with good comprehension of what has been read. In some patients, however, reading comprehension may be impaired while auditory comprehension is retained, a finding that suggests additional involvement beyond the pure syndrome of conduction aphasia.

The ability to write is invariably disturbed to some degree in conduction aphasia. Most often the patient can write some words and produce well-formed letters but the spelling is poor, with omissions, reversals and substitutions of letters. Words in a sentence are frequently interchanged, misplaced or omitted. The examiner may be able to guess the intended meaning but the output is far from acceptable.

In many instances, conduction aphasia cannot be diagnosed at the onset but develops during the course of recovery. Most often such a patient will originally produce a severe neologistic jargon and show considerable comprehension deficit. As the condition improves, the jargon clears to literal paraphasia and there is a concomitant improvement in auditory comprehension leading to the cluster of symptoms called conduction aphasia. The improvement often continues and many individuals with a disorder called conduction aphasia eventually have only an anomia.

The neurologic examination in conduction aphasia has considerable variation. Often almost no neurologic abnormality can be demonstrated. Others, however, suffer considerable elementary neurologic abnormality. Unilateral paresis may be totally absent, mildly present or significant. The weakness almost always involves the arm to a greater degree than the leg. Sensory findings are also variable, from totally absent to a limited sensory loss. Individual cases have been recorded with cortical sensory loss limited to the dominant upper extremity, some only having involvement of the index and middle fingers, suggesting a small but precise lesion involving the parietal-sensory cortex or pathways between the thalamus and the sensory cortex. Late in recovery from conduction aphasia a rather specific pain syndrome may be present. This has been called the "pseudothalamic pain syndrome" to suggest a resemblance but distinct difference when compared to the classic thalamic pain syndrome. The pain is constant but of a less intense degree and is not exacerbated by external stimuli. It has been suggested that the pseudothalamic pain syndrome occurs following separation of the thalamic nuclei from the parietal operculum (S II area). These patients have a combination of cortical sensory loss, decreased pain realization plus paresthesias and hyperalgesia. In contrast, some individuals with conduction aphasia have *pain asymbolia* (Biemond, 1956; Geschwind, 1965). In this situation, the patient appears to respond to pain stimuli considerably less than anticipated. The decreased realization of pain is bilateral even though the pathology is limited to the left hemisphere. While a bilateral decrease in pain response cannot be found in all, some patients with conduction aphasia do appear to tolerate more pain than other patients.

There is also a considerable variation in the findings on examination of the visual system in conduction aphasia. While there is usually no involvement of extraocular movement, the visual fields are frequently abnormal. The variations are complete; some show no visual field defect, others have a full hemianopsia, some show upper and others lower quadrantanopsia. The extreme variability probably reflects involvement of different sites neighboring the locus of pathology underlying conduction aphasia.

Ideomotor apraxia is frequently but not constantly present. When asked to perform bucco-facial or limb movements on command the patient may fail, even while protesting that he knows what he wants to do. Just as often the result is an improper movement which nevertheless demonstrates comprehension of the command (such as waving the hand near the face when asked to salute); the ability to imitate the movement is intact. The incorrect, extraneous movements on command appear to parallel the paraphasia which contaminates the repetition. Not all patients with conduction aphasia show ideomotor apraxia, however, and the distinction appears to have anatomical bearing.

Conduction aphasia has been localized by CT scan (Naeser and Hayward, 1978) radioisotope brain scan (Kertesz, Lesk and McCabe, 1977) and pathological studies (Kleist, 1934; Benson et al, 1973). The lesion in conduction aphasia is limited in size, the smallest among the major varieties of aphasia, making demonstration somewhat difficult. Negative results are not infrequent but many cases have been recorded with firm evidence concerning the location of pathology in conduction aphasia.

Pathologically, several clinical entities are known to produce conduction aphasia. The most common, of course, is cerebral vascular accident, most often occlusion of a portion of the angular branch of the middle cerebral artery.

Both tumor (Brown, 1972) and trauma (often a traumatic intracerebral hematoma) are recognized as sources of this disorder. It is not the pathology, however, but the site of the lesion that produces the unique combination of language functions.

The site of pathology in conduction aphasia, however, shows some variation. Two distinctly different locations have been demonstrated (Lichtheim, 1885; Kleist, 1934b; Hecaen, Dell and Roger, 1955; Benson et al, 1973). One involves the dominant hemisphere arcuate fasciculus, a band of white matter originating in the posterior temporal lobe and coursing forward via the superior longitudinal fasciculus to the motor association cortex of the frontal lobe (see Fig. 7-4). Involvement of the arcuate fasciculus, most often deep in the supramarginal gyrus, could produce the separation of the sensory and motor language areas originally suggested by Wernicke. Involvement of the arcuate fasciculus has been proved in a number of cases of conduction aphasia studied at postmortem but some authorities insist that involvement of the supramarginal cortex, not the underlying white matter, is the essential finding. This disagreement remains unsettled. In addition to this suprasylvian site, however, a number of reports of conduction aphasia demonstrate that pathology in a subsylvian locus, specifically involvement of the dominant auditory association cortex (Wernicke's area) can be the cause. On this basis Kleist (1934b) conjectured that some patients comprehend spoken language with the right hemisphere but only speak with the left motor language area. If this is true, a lesion destroying the dominant auditory association area could disconnect the areas which carry out language comprehension (right hemisphere) from the motor speech area (left hemisphere) and produce the syndrome of conduction aphasia (good comprehension and fluent output but inability to repeat) (see Fig. 7-5). While the location of the lesion in conduction aphasia is not fixed, all agree that when the clinical syndrome of conduction aphasia is demonstrated, pathology will be located somewhere in the posterior sylvian region, either above, below or behind the end of the dominant sylvian fissure.

Finally, it should be noted that in one report (Benson et al, 1973) the combination of ideomotor apraxia and conduction aphasia was present in individuals with suprasylvian pathology (involving the arcuate fasciculus) while conduction aphasia without apraxia was present with subsylvian location of the pathology. This observation was consistent with reports in the literature but there are too few cases to allow final decision. Despite the well-documented disagreement on the location of pathology, the syndrome of conduction aphasia is fully recognizable, occurs rather commonly and offers excellent localizing information for the clinician.

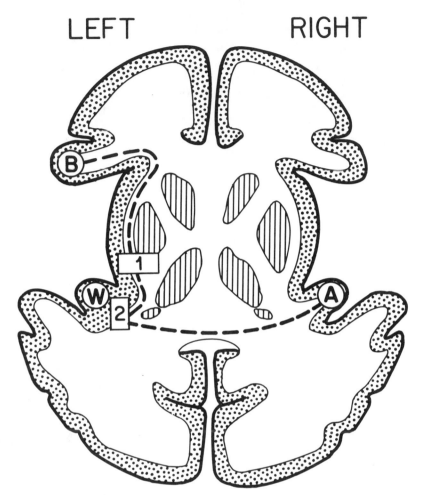

LEFT   **RIGHT**

Figure 7-5. *Highly schematic horizontal section showing the two sites of pathology in conduction aphasia suggested by Kleist. "A" represents the right temporal auditory association cortes, W = Wernicke's area, B = Broca's area, 1 = Site of arcuate fasciculus pathology and 2 = Wernicke's area pathology; both 1 and 2 have been suggested as sites of pathology in conduction aphasia.*

8

Borderzone Aphasic Syndromes

The clinical feature common to all three of the aphasia syndromes described in the last chapter was defective repetition of spoken language, and the common neuroanatomical feature was pathological involvement of the perisylvian speech area. Although less common in pure states, there are a number of aphasia syndromes in which repetition remains normal or considerably superior to other language functions. Almost without exception the aphasia syndromes without repetition disturbance indicate pathology located outside the perisylvian region. The area involved is located in the vascular borderzone between the territory of the middle cerebral artery and those of the anterior or posterior cerebral arteries (Fig. 3-4). Clinical variation in these syndromes can usually be correlated with the portion of the borderzone involved. The term *transcortical aphasia* was suggested by Wernicke (1881) and Lichtheim (1885) and this group of aphasia syndromes was intensely studied by Goldstein (1917). The term transcortical aphasia originally contrasted the aphasias with retained repetition with cortical and subcortical varieties in a postulated anatomical model of language and ideation which has long been abandoned. As Goldstein noted, the term transcortical is archaic, but when used only to identify those aphasic syndromes sharing the feature of retained ability to repeat spoken language, it retains a usefulness. Other terms have been proposed for these aphasia syndromes, mostly derived from later models of language function that are just as suspect as the original theories. Transcortical remains the most widely used and generally accepted term for delineating this group of aphasic syndromes.

Both the term transcortical aphasia and the separable aphasic syndromes included under this term were out of favor for many years, but in recent years they have been returned to acceptance and are now reported in a sizable number of studies. There are many suggestions as to why repetition is spared in aphasia, again usually based on unsupported theories of language function such as Lichtheim's.

TRANSCORTICAL MOTOR APHASIA

A number of names have been suggested for this variety of aphasia including *dynamic aphasia* (Luria, 1966) and *anterior isolation syndrome* (Benson and Geschwind, 1971), but *transcortical motor aphasia*, the term suggested by Lichtheim, has the widest acceptance. Goldstein (1948) postulated that two different problems could produce this syndrome. One was a partial recovery from Broca aphasia in which repetition as a function was recovered better than the ability to speak spontaneously. His second variation was the result of a primary difficulty in initiation of the articulatory process, corrected by prompting. Transcortical motor aphasia has a number of definitive findings that are outlined in Table 8-1.

Table 8-1. BASIC LANGUAGE CHARACTERISTICS OF TRANSCORTICAL MOTOR APHASIA

Conversational speech	Nonfluent
Comprehension of spoken language	Relatively normal
Repetition of spoken language	Good to fully normal
Confrontation-naming	Defective
Reading: Aloud	Defective
Comprehension	Often Good
Writing	Defective

While the spontaneous speech of transcortical motor aphasia (TCM) can be described as nonfluent, the output characteristics differ from those of Broca aphasia. Dysarthria may be severe in both but in TCM there is more tendency for a stumbling, repetitive, even stuttering spontaneous output. Often the same poorly articulated syllable or group of syllables will be repeated many times in an attempt to respond. Conversational verbalization is almost invariably agrammatic, highly simplified and produced with considerable effort. A dramatic output feature seen in many is the patient's attempt to use motor prompting to initiate speech. Patients with TCM have been noted to direct themselves with their hands (like a symphony conductor) or to stand up and sit down, using each motion to aid initiation of a word. TCM patients have been described who could only initiate a syllable or word as the left foot struck the ground during walking and had learned to pace back and forth to prompt their verbal output. While there is considerable variation in the difficulty a TCM aphasic has in verbal output, this is almost always a striking abnormality.

Series speech, on the other hand, is performed surprisingly well once the series in initiated. If a TCM patient who fails to count on request is given the first one or two numbers, the series is often continued unhindered, at least for a time. Similarly, recitation of nursery rhymes, names of the days or months, etc. are often successfully performed if started by the examiner. When the task is failed, it is often directly attributable to perseveration, an inability to halt the continuous repetition of a single word.

Comprehension of spoken language usually appears good, at least in normal conversation. Patients with transcortical motor aphasia often have difficulty handling sequences of material and some have difficulty understanding specific relational words (i.e. larger-smaller, in-out, etc.) just as in Broca aphasia. Comprehension can prove difficult to test in patients with transcortical motor aphasia also. They may have difficulty in controlling yes-no responses, contamination by perseveration is common and production of meaningless responses can be seen. Similarly apraxia is often severe in TCM so that the patient may neither point to room objects readily nor carry out commands. Tests must be devised for these patients individually to demonstrate the considerable retention of spoken language comprehension.

Repetition is the most striking feature of this syndrome. The ability to repeat is always unexpectedly good and may be truly excellent. TCM patients may echo a word or phrase but they usually are not truly echolalic in the fashion of a mandatory repetition. They will correct grammatically incorrect statements they are asked to repeat and will reject nonsense syllables and grammatically incorrect statements. A strong demonstration of the completion phenomenon is common; if a nursery rhyme, poem or overlearned statement is started by the examiner it can be completed easily and almost automatically by the patient.

The ability to produce names on confrontation is often limited. Again, the patient shows problems in initiating articulation and produces repetitious sounds in a manner similar to that noted in spontaneous conversation. With judicious prompting, TCM patients often show dramatic improvement in their ability to name. Either contextual cues or phonemic cues may be helpful but the former often appear most useful. Not always, however, is the entire problem in confrontation-naming a problem of articulation. Even with prompting, TCM patients may fail to name, and even more strikingly they may produce incorrect words if given incorrect cues. Thus, true problems in word-finding must be suspected in these patients.

Almost invariably, TCM patients have difficulty reading out loud, producing a poorly articulated output. On the other hand, the comprehension of written material is often good. In general, comprehension of written material is better in patients with transcortical motor aphasia than in those with Broca aphasia. There are exceptions, however, and some patients with TCM show a significant alexia with appropriate testing.

The ability to write is almost universally defective, often seriously, in transcortical motor aphasia. The written language output features large, clumsily produced letters, poor spelling and hypereconomic or agrammatic output.

The neighborhood findings in transcortical motor aphasia are, in general, similar to those present in Broca aphasia. Most TCM patients have right hemiplegia although this is not a mandatory finding. Similarly, apraxia is extremely common so that not only is the right side paralyzed but TCM patients often fail to use the left limbs correctly for verbally directed activities. Neither sensory loss nor visual field loss is characteristic but both are seen occasionally, dependent upon the size and site of the lesion. The presence of conjugate deviation and unilateral inattention syndrome (see Ch. 16) in the initial stages of transcortical motor aphasia has been recorded in some but not all.

The course of transcortical motor aphasia has not been as well recorded as have some other varieties of aphasia. Some investigators continue to believe that TCM represents a stage in recovery from a more profound motor aphasia, not a separate disorder. Others assert that transcortical motor aphasia represents a portion of the total Broca aphasia picture and that patients with transcortical motor aphasia have an incomplete form of Broca aphasia. Our own experience suggests that the recovery from transcortical motor aphasia is rather limited and patients with TCM have proved difficult to treat. Others (Rubens, 1976; Kertesz and McCabe, 1977), however, report considerable recovery, with and without treatment, in selected patients with transcortical motor aphasia.

Transcortical motor aphasia has proved rather easy to demonstrate with readioisotope studies (Rubens, 1976; Kertesz, Lesk and McCabe, 1977), CT scan (Naeser and Hayward, 1978) and EEG (Alexander and Schmitt, 1979). The location of surgical pathology, both tumor excision and trauma, has also proved useful for localizing purposes in cases with TCM.

Transcortical motor aphasia may be produced by a wide variety of pathologies. One of the more striking is tumor, particularly a frontal glioma that has been radically excised. TCM may occur following occlusive vascular disease but is probably more common as a result of intracerebral hematoma than with either thrombotic or embolic disease. More distant occlusive disease, specifically acute occlusion of the internal carotid artery in the neck producing a borderzone area infarction, is one of the more common causes. Recent case reports (Rubens, 1976; DeMasio and Kassel, 1978) document occlusion of the dominant anterior cerebral artery causing medial-frontal infarction in individuals who show classic TCM findings. Trauma, most notably gunshot wound to the appropriate area of the brain, can also produce this particular symptom constellation.

The striking specificity of the transcortical motor aphasia syndrome appears linked to the specific site or sites of pathology. Almost without exception, cases with the features of transcortical motor aphasia will have pathology located either anterior to or superior to Broca's area in the dominant frontal lobe. Most characteristically, the pathology involves the middle or anterior portions of the third frontal gyrus, the second or possibly even the first frontal gyrus. In addition, there are occasional reports of this language syndrome following infarction in the anterior cerebral artery territory (see below), but the pathology always involves the dominant frontal lobe somewhere exclusive of Broca's area.

APHASIA FOLLOWING ANTERIOR CEREBRAL ARTERY OCCLUSION

Critchley (1930) reviewed the anatomical and clinical aspects of anterior cerebral artery occlusion and noted that aphasia was an occasional finding. In the style of the day, the type of language disturbance was not defined. Recently, Rubens (1976) described the aphasia syndrome in two individuals following acute occlusion of the dominant (left) anterior cerebral artery. The speech and language features included: 1) an initial period of mutism lasting 2 and 10 days respectively leading to 2) a transient aphasia featuring almost total inability to initiate speech in contrast to 3) nearly intact repetition, 4) no phonemic paraphasia, 5) essentially normal comprehension and confrontation-naming and 6) neither echolalia nor forced completion phenomenon. While reading aloud was at a near-normal level, reading comprehension was limited to object-picture matching. Both patients manifested distinct trouble in the comprehension of relational, syntactical linguistic structures. It was concluded that the aphasia syndrome in these two individuals most closely resembled the transcortical motor aphasia syndrome. Two recent reports (DeMasio and Kassel, 1978; Alexander and Schmitt, 1979) corroborate Rubens' findings with additional case material.

The neighborhood neurologic findings with anterior cerebral artery occlusion are notable. Profound weakness, hyperreflexia, extensor toe signs and sensory loss are present in the right lower extremity with a mild weakness of the right shoulder but excellent arm, hand and face strength and no other neurologic involvement. These are the classic neurologic findings of infarction involving the anterior cerebral artery territory (Fisher, 1975) and this localization was confirmed in all cases by either radioactive isotope brain scans or CT scans. Rubens' patients showed considerable recovery of language over a period of several months. Aphasia secondary to left anterior cerebral artery occlusion is not common but appears to result in a clinical syndrome similar or identical to that called transcortical motor aphasia.

TRANSCORTICAL SENSORY APHASIA

Historically, the demonstration of transcortical sensory aphasia (TCS) can also be traced to the work of Lichtheim and Wernicke who originally postulated that this specific language syndrome occurred following disconnection of the sensory language area and the "concept area." Their theory has not been accepted but many investigators have noted this variety of aphasia including Bastian (1898), Pick (1931) and others. Most often, the investigators were originally fascinated by the phenomenon of echolalia and in many discussions of transcortical sensory aphasia, echolalia is the only language process discussed, almost as though echolalia represented a specific aphasia syndrome. Goldstein, in his major study of transcortical aphasia (1917), clearly outlined and described the features of transcortical sensory aphasia but devoted most of the discussion to the phenomena of repetition and echolalia. The clinical features of TCS listed in Table 8-2 are quite distinct and worthy of clinical attention.

The conversational speech in transcortical sensory aphasia is unquestionably fluent, often contaminated by considerable paraphasia, including both neologistic and semantic substitutions, and frequently features a notable emptiness. The most striking quality, however, is *echolalia* (see Ch. 4). TCS patients almost routinely incorporate words and phrases uttered by the examiner into their own ongoing output while apparently failing to respond to the meaning of these words. In TCS the echolalia often appears mandatory, the patient

Table 8-2. BASIC LANGUAGE CHARACTERISTICS OF
TRANSCORTICAL SENSORY APHASIA

Conversational speech	Fluent, paraphasic, echolalic
Comprehension of spoken language	Severely defective
Repetition of spoken language	Good to excellent
Confrontation-naming	Defective
Reading: Aloud	Defective
Comprehension	Defective
Writing	Defective

apparently unable to omit the examiner's words. Incorrect syntactical structures, nonsense words and even foreign phrases may be echoed. The total
output is often verbose, with a tendency to run on almost uninhibited. Series
speech, if initiated by the examiner, is notably good. TCS patients can count
and recite the days and months, and the completion phenomenon for poems
and statements (see Ch. 4) is usually very strong.

Comprehension of spoken language is severely disturbed in TCS often to
the point of total noncomprehension, and offers a dramatic contrast to the ease
with which the examiner's statements are reiterated. Many TCS patients completely fail all attempts to demonstrate understanding of spoken language including pointing tasks, carrying out commands and answering yes/no questions. Obviously, there are gradations of the severity of comprehension disturbance in TCS. Some claim that TCS and anomic aphasia are on a spectrum,
with a severe comprehension defect in TCS, excellent comprehension in
anomic aphasia and patients with partial ability to comprehend placed in one or
the other categories at the discretion of the observer.

In striking contrast to the severe comprehension defect, repetition of utterances ranges from good to excellent. The span level for auditory material may
be somewhat low and limit the overall ability to repeat but even the span is
remarkably good in many cases. The TCS patient tends to repeat absolutely
and accurately what is said and, as noted, will often repeat nonsense syllables,
Jabberwocky, foreign phrases and grammatically incorrect utterances verbatim
and with apparent unawareness of what is said.

Naming is seriously defective in TCS. Characteristically, these patients
neither name an object nor identify an object when the name is given. At times
TCS patients offer names which are incorrect but they are even more likely to
present a long, unrelated sentence which fails to describe the item.

While not constant, the ability to read aloud may be preserved in patients
with transcortical sensory aphasia. Reading for comprehension, on the other
hand, is almost invariably seriously defective so that even those who can read
aloud with accuracy fail to understand what they have just said (just as they fail
to comprehend spoken language that they repeat flawlessly). Very often, however, TCS patients make paraphasic substitutions when reading aloud. Words,
or even entire phrases, may be substituted during attempts to read out loud.

Writing is defective and, in general, shows features similar to the disturbance of written output seen with Wernicke aphasia.

TCS patients may show some degree of paresis but this tends to be mild and transient or entirely absent. Sensory abnormality is often present but may be mild and may be restricted to a mild cortical sensory abnormality. Visual field defect is frequently present but may be a superior quandrantanopsia, inferior quadrantanopsia, full hemianopic defect or some in-between stage. Some patients with transcortical sensory aphasia have no obvious elementary neurologic deficit.

As could be anticipated, TCS patients with excellent ability to repeat a question but unable to understand it and showing no neurologic deficit are easily misdiagnosed as psychotic. Many of the most striking examples of TCS observed by the author have been patients maintained in mental hospitals with a diagnosis of schizophrenia.

Transcortical sensory aphasia has not been as widely recognized as the other disorders discussed and there are less accumulated data on the ability to localize the pathology. Kertesz, Lesk and McCabe (1977) report three cases of TCS with focal lesions demonstrated by radioisotope scan. CT scanning, surgical excisions and focal brain injury have all been used to localize TCS but the accumulated data are too small to warrant claims of accuracy.

Transcortical sensory aphasia often begins with a global disturbance including limited output and no comprehension. Next a state of neologistic jargon evolves featuring a considerable output of almost unconnected syllables with a decrease in the neologistic paraphasia, much of the output consists of real words or meaningful phrases which bear no relationship to the examiner's statement. At this stage, a superb ability to repeat can be demonstrated. The prognosis in TCS is usually guarded although there is some tendency for improvement in the comprehension of spoken language. Kertesz and McCabe (1977) consider TCS to have an excellent prognosis.

A number of pathological disorders can produce transcortical sensory aphasia. The most common cause is vascular disease, particularly occlusive disease of the great vessels. Occlusion of the left internal carotid artery with a subsequent posterior borderzone infarction frequently underlies transcortical sensory aphasia and should be suspected whenever the syndrome is present. Tumors in the parietal-temporal-occipital junction area can produce this syndrome and trauma is reported as a common cause by Kertesz and McCabe (1977). Intracerebral hematoma is an uncommon but recognized cause of TCS.

The site of pathological lesion in transcortical sensory aphasia is even less exact than that of transcortical motor aphasia. While invariably posterior, the lesion may involve either the parietal borderzone, the temporal borderzone or a combination of these areas (see Fig. 8-1). Frequently transcortical sensory aphasia is seen with sizeable pathological lesions and evolves from rather messy symptom pictures. Well-defined pictures of transcortical sensory aphasia are not common. That the syndrome does exist, however, is definite and the location of pathology in the best defined cases has involved the posterior temporal-parietal junction area of the dominant hemisphere.

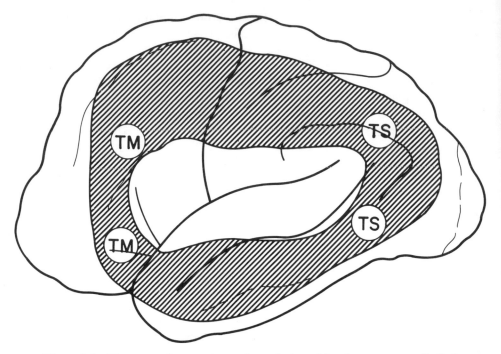

Figure 8-1. Diagram of approximate boundaries of borderzone area. Pathology is present in the lined area but not in the inner language area in most instances of borderzone aphasia. *TM* = possible sites of transcortical motor aphasia; *TS* = possible sites for transcortical sensory aphasia. Involvement of borderzone area both anteriorly and posteriorly underlies the mixed transcortical aphasia picture.

MIXED TRANSCORTICAL APHASIA
(ISOLATION OF THE SPEECH AREA)

This fascinating variety of aphasia, rare in pure form but occasionally noted in less exact circumstances, has been well-described and thoroughly discussed (Goldstein, 1917, 1948; Geschwind, Quadfasel and Segarra, 1968; Whitaker, 1976b). While not common, study of the mixed transcortical syndrome provides meaningful insights to the anatomical bases of certain language functions and the well-studied cases that include autopsy correlation are of considerable significance. Two names have been suggested for this syndrome. One, *isolation of the speech area,* emphasizes the clinical picture. The second, *mixed transcortical aphasia,* recognizes that there is a combination of the features of the transcortical motor and transcortical sensory syndromes. The clinical characteristics are almost unbelievable, even more striking than indicated by Table 8-3. Most dramatically, only repetition is preserved of all the language functions.

Patients with mixed transcortical aphasia (MTA) do not speak unless spo-

Table 8-3. BASIC LANGUAGE CHARACTERISTICS OF
MIXED TRANSCORTICAL APHASIA

Conversational speech	Nonfluent with echolalia
Comprehension of spoken language	Severely defective
Repetition of spoken language	Good
Confrontation-naming	Severely defective
Reading: Aloud	Defective
Comprehension	Defective
Writing	Defective

ken to and then their verbal output is almost entirely limited to what has been offered by the examiner, a true echolalia. The patient with MTA may, however, embellish the output somewhat, particularly in the form of the completion phenomenon. Thus, if told the beginning of a common phrase, the patient may not only repeat what has been said but continue the phrase to completion. Articulation is surprisingly clear. Series speech is comparatively good once the patient is started on the task. Thus if started to count, to give names of the days or months or to recite nursery rhymes or poems, the patient can often continue the activity with ease. If interrupted, however, the patient cannot continue and there is a feeling that the response is automatic, not done with understanding, similar to the reading of a passage from a noncomprehended language.

Comprehension of spoken language is severely disturbed in MTA. In the most classic cases described in the literature there has been absolutely no evidence of comprehension of spoken language. Some cases we have observed clinically have had some degree of comprehension ability demonstrated on some occasions but comprehension has always been extremely limited.

The ability to repeat, while dramatically preserved compared to all other language features, remains limited and is often well below normal. The number of words in a phrase that can be repeated is often limited to just three or four. As already noted, MTA patients show the characteristics of the completion phenomenon. They will complete common sentences or phrases, may or may not correct grammatically incorrect phrases and they repeat nonsense syllables and foreign words quite accurately. All of these tasks are limited, however, by the short span.

Patients with the true mixed transcortical aphasia syndrome have severe difficulty in naming, sometimes producing neologisms or semantic paraphasias but frequently producing no response at all. Similarly, the ability to read out loud, the ability to comprehend what is read and the ability to write are severely disturbed in this disorder. In elementary terms, the patient with a mixed transcortical aphasia has a global aphasia except for the dramatic preservation of the ability to repeat what has been said.

The neurologic findings in the few cases of this disorder that have been adequately reported have been quite variable. Several of the cases have shown bilateral upper motor neuron paralysis producing a severe spastic quadriparesis. Other cases have unilateral motor disturbance, right hemiplegia, plus a significant sensory loss. A visual field defect, usually a right homonymous hemianopia, has been present in the few cases reported. The mixed transcortical syndrome appears to occur only in individuals with severe brain damage. There are very few reports of localizing techniques in MTA and none are exact except for autopsy. It could be anticipated that both the isotope brain scan and the CT scan would demonstrate severe and widespread pictures of cerebral involvement.

The course of mixed transcortical aphasia appears to be stable but unimproving. Most patients with the syndrome reported in the literature and those seen in our clinic have shown little tendency for recovery. In addition to the few classic case studies in the literature which showed little significant improvement, Kertesz and McCabe (1977) report two cases of "isolation syndrome" that improved only slightly and the author has cared for three individuals with MTA, all of whom improved to only a minimal degree. The total number of cases reported is far too small, however, to hazard specific predictions in any individual with MTA.

Despite the limited number of cases recorded in the literature and seen personally, a suprising variety of pathology has been reported. The case of Geschwind et al was secondary to self-inflicted anoxia. Goldstein recorded five cases from the early literature showing the characteristics of MTA; two had suffered major cerebral vascular insults while the other three had diffuse encephalopathy, in two with superimposed left hemisphere pathology. One case observed by the author was the result of cerebral edema following trauma to the brain. Two other cases had suffered acute carotid occlusion, apparently producing a total borderzone infarction. Each variety of pathology described has produced a fairly wide field of pathology. The most intense involvement, however, has been proved or presumed to be in the vascular borderzone of the dominant hemisphere. The case of hypoxia studied at postmortem (Geschwind, Quadfasel and Segarra, 1968) showed rather exact localization of the pathology to the borderzone areas. Similarly, both the carotid occlusion and cerebral edema etiologies can be conjectured to produce decreased cerebral oxygen supply having a maximal impact on the borderzone area. Thus, the syndrome of mixed transcortical aphasia strongly suggests a locus of pathology involving the cerebral vascular borderzone (see Fig. 8-1).

9

Subcortical Aphasic Syndromes

Most of the aphasic syndromes outlined in the previous two chapters have been described and discussed for many years. A considerable body of clinical-neuroanatomical correlation has become available and each syndrome appears fairly well established as a clinical entity. Nonetheless, every clinician realizes that the features in many individuals with aphasia fail to truly match any one of these syndromes. At the same time, when appropriate studies are performed, many aphasics have pathology outside the anticipated locale. One obvious explanation for the many nonclassic aphasics rests on the purely cortical localization usually suggested for the classic syndromes. It has long been accepted that the classic syndromes were probably the products of combined cortical and subcortical involvement but there has been little recognition that aphasia could result from subcortical pathology alone, nor have there been any accepted descriptions of aphasic syndromes secondary to subcortical involvement.

Recent technological advances, particularly improved pharmacologic and nursing treatment for intracerebral hemorrhage and the availability of CAT scans, have suddenly provided frequent delineation of subcortical pathology in the living patient. Rethinking of the previously hypothesized effects of subcortical damage to language has been necessary and new aphasia syndromes, based on purely subcortical damage, have been suggested. Most often the newly noted types of subcortical language disturbance follow acute intracerebral hemorrhage. Almost without exception, language problems have occurred only when left hemisphere structures (thalamus, striatum, claustrum, insula) have been involved. Alterations in speech, beginning with mutism and followed by hypophonia, slow, sparse output and poorly differentiated, amelodic articulation are described and resemble, at least superficially, the verbal output that often complicated thalamotomy for the treatment of parkinsonism (Riklan and Levita, 1970). Language defects are less specific but several features, particularly the combination of a severely paraphasic output contrasted with comparatively normal repetition appear to present a distinct pattern.

The syndromes to be described here must be considered tentative and will deserve reconsideration as additional clinical observations become available. Whether these syndromes actually represent the effects of subcortical pathology or merely the distant effects of an acutely produced, deep mass lesion remains an unsettled question. Nonetheless, certain types of subcortical pathology appear to affect language function and deserve consideration in the pathology of language, both as separate entities and as complicating factors for the classic cortical aphasic syndromes.

THE APHASIA OF MARIE'S QUADRILATERAL SPACE

One variety of subcortical aphasia has a long but controversial history and probably represents a greater reality than often admitted. The aphasia of Marie's quadrilateral space has been the source of deep argument, either accepted or rejected by proponents or opponents, respectively, of the holistic approach to aphasia. When Marie suggested that the aphasia described by Broca was not a true aphasia (1906), some of his contemporaries considered it an heretical, almost blasphemous statement. In defense of his position Marie proposed that patients with "Broca's aphasia" consistently had pathology occupying the area deep to the insula (Island of Reil) in a space subsequently known as Marie's quadrilateral space (see Fig. 9-1). He noted that the two cases originally cited by Broca had pathology involving this anatomical area in addition to the traditionally described posterior-inferior frontal cortex damage. Marie went on to suggest that the only true aphasia was Wernicke aphasia (a disturbance of language comprehension) and that pathology in the quadrilateral space did not, by itself, produce aphasia. What was produced was a severe disturbance of verbal output that Marie called *anarthria.* For a patient with pathology in Broca's area to be truly aphasic, the pathology had to extend posteriorly to involve Wernicke's area or its connections to the thalamus. Marie's suggestion produced heated debate and still has both opponents and adherents. The recent demonstration of unique problems in comprehension and expression involving the syntactical, grammatical constructions of language in patients with Broca aphasia (Zurif, Caramazza and Myerson, 1972; Samuels and Benson, 1979) appears to disprove Marie's suggestion that Broca aphasia is not a specific language disturbance. These linguistic findings are newly demonstrated, however; they are still not widely recognized and demand replication. Many aphasiologists continue to respect and promote Marie's postulate of a single aphasia and believe that aphasics suffering destruction restricted to Marie's quadrilateral space and/or Broca's area are anarthric, not aphasic.

From a purely observational viewpoint, excluding the theoretical discussions, many individuals are seen whose aphasia is neither Broca aphasia nor Wernicke aphasia and who have pathology involving the quadrilateral space. Unfortunately, Marie did not offer a precise clinical picture for the aphasia resulting from pathology involving the quadrilateral space, and to date the available descriptions are sketchy. Pathology involving this area (almost always a deep hemorrhage) produces acute mutism and a dense right hemiplegia. With improvement a nonfluent aphasia with greater or lesser degrees of comprehension difficulty develops. In Marie's view, the presence of aphasia, as demonstrated by language comprehension defect, would indicate posterior extension of the lesion to involve the temporal isthmus. In current terminology many such cases (featuring a dense nonfluent output and significant com-

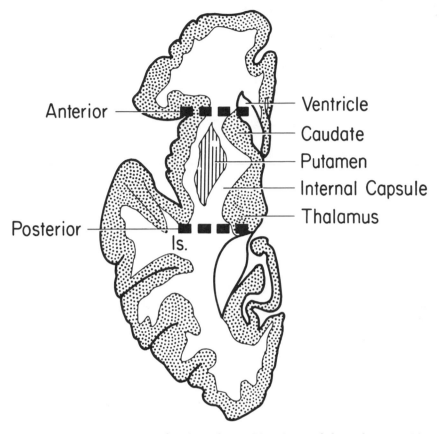

Figure 9-1. *Diagrammatic sketch outlining Marie's quadrilateral space. The heavy broken lines indicate the anterior and posterior boundaries of the space. Destruction of tissue posteriorly, particularly involving the temporal isthmus (Is.), was considered necessary to produce a true (Wernicke) aphasia.*

prehension defect) would be called global aphasia. Lesser amounts of destruction of this area undoubtedly exist, and if the pathology primarily destroys specific areas, either a striatal or a thalamic aphasia syndrome can be postulated (see below). If, as frequently occurs, the structural destruction extends anteriorly and superficially, involving both Marie's quadrilateral space and Broca's area, Broca aphasia may result.

Another specific disturbance of verbal function may be postulated as indicating destruction in the quadrilateral space but avoiding Broca's area and most of the putamen and thalamus. When severe articulatory disturbance (slow, hypophonic, amelodic, breathy verbalization) is the predominant verbal abnormality in a patient following a left hemisphere destructive lesion, Marie's anarthria and anterior subcortical localization can be suspected. At present there is insufficient case material to support this conjecture and future clinical-neuroanatomical correlations particularly utilizing the CAT scan, will be necessary to provide confirmation or denial. Nonetheless, that a specific syndrome indicating involvement of Marie's quadrilateral space in the dominant hemisphere could exist seems entirely possible, and that destruction of this area in combination with cortical language areas could produce more complex language syndromes would appear highly probable.

THALAMIC APHASIA

For many years a debate has raged over the role the dominant thalamus plays in aphasia. As recently as 1968, an entire mechanism of aphasia was proposed that was based on pathology involving the thalamic pulvinar with extension to various cortical regions (J. R. Brown, 1968) and a number of reports documenting thalamic involvement in individuals with significant language disturbance have appeared (Penfield and Roberts, 1959; Van Buren and Burke, 1969; Ciemins, 1970). On the other hand, other studies have insisted that thalamic pathology does not produce aphasia. In particular, follow-up studies of patients who underwent thalamic destruction for treatment of movement disorder demonstrate little alteration in language (Dubois et al, 1966; Riklan and Levita, 1970; J. W. Brown, 1974; Van Buren, 1975). While aphasia following thalamic destruction appears to be very rare, the impossibility of proving a negative has kept the controversy alive. With the introduction of the CAT scan in the past few years additional information has become available. This instrument is far better at demonstrating deep hemorrhage than any previous technique and a growing number of cases of thalamic hemorrhage are being published (Ciemins, 1970; Mohr, Watters and Duncan, 1975; Samarel et al, 1976; Luria, 1977) with discussion on the occurrence of aphasia. Most indicate that left thalamic damage produces an aphasia but some deny a direct relationship of the thalamus to language.

Thalamic hemorrhage usually produces an acute, catastrophic picture with hemiplegia, hemisensory loss, right visual field defect and alteration of the level of consciousness, often to the degree of coma. The original language abnormality is mutism, or near-mutism, but eventually this changes to a verbose paraphasic, jargon output. Anomia is often severe, almost a total failure to name on confrontation, but, differing dramatically from other fluent paraphasic syndromes with serious anomia, individuals with thalamic hemorrhage show comparatively good comprehension and an unanticipated competency at repeating spoken language. Reading and writing are usually disturbed to a significant degree although not as severely as in many cases of posterior aphasia or alexia with agraphia. The language findings following thalamic hemorrhage tend to be transient, a most significant finding. Recovery often begins within days or weeks and, except in cases complicated by widespread damage, the course is usually one of consistent improvement over a period of a few weeks or months. Recovery from paresis is even more rapid but some degree of hemisensory abnormality often remains. Clinically, the combination of logorrheic, paraphasic output, comparatively good comprehension and unexpectedly good repetition can be considered suggestive of posterior subcortical aphasia. Confirmation is best derived from the CAT scan (see Fig. 9-2). It should be remembered that while the prognosis for the aphasia of thalamic hematoma is generally good, the same is not true of the causative disorder. Many individuals with intracerebral hemorrhage never recover sufficiently to allow evaluation of the aphasia and the mortality rate remains high (Lishman, 1978). Not all individuals with left thalamic hemorrhage recover completely and the role of the dominant hemisphere thalamus in language remains unsettled.

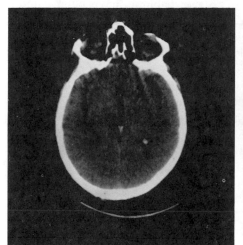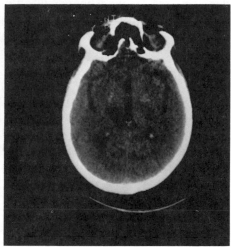

Figure 9-2. CAT scan (2 views) demonstrating a small, punched out, lucent area indicating the site of an old hemorrhage in the left thalamus. Originally the patient was mute, then hypophonic, paraphasic and anomic but had recovered language function by the time this scan was performed.

The existence of "thalamic aphasia" as an entity remains controversial. Impressed by the wealth of thalamo-cortical connections, some investigators promote a major language function for the thalamus and accept the syndrome described above as a primary variety of aphasia indicating thalamic damage. Support for this stance stems from a number of sources, not the least of which is the direct clinical-pathological observation of thalamic damage associated with aphasia. A primary language function for the thalamus receives additional support from the production of aphasic elements (paraphasia and anomia) with electrical stimulation of the left pulvinar (Ojemann and Ward, 1971; Fedio and Van Buren, 1975). Other investigators, however, point out that most individuals suffer no permanent aphasia despite severe thalamic damage, and they suggest that the aphasia following thalamic hemorrhage is a variant of transcortical sensory aphasia secondary to borderzone ischemia, caused by a deep source of greatly increased pressure. Whichever theory is correct, there seems little doubt that left thalamic hemorrhage is frequently associated with a language abnormality, and that it often has distinctive features and deserves separate consideration. An extreme paradox appears to be present, a distinct lanquage defect syndrome that deserves the name thalamic aphasia in the face of strong evidence that thalamic damage does not lead to permanent language defect.

STRIATAL APHASIA

With the use of the CAT scan individual cases of intracerebral hematoma deep in the left hemisphere but anterior to the thalamus have been demonstrated. With retrospective speculation it appears that a separate aphasic syndrome might follow acute hemorrhage restricted to the putamen-caudate-globus pallidus area of the left hemisphere. Very few cases of "striatal" aphasia have been recorded but from several cases observed personally, and others described by colleagues, a language syndrome can be postulated.

As with all intracerebral hemorrhagic syndromes, striatal hematoma begins acutely, usually with a severe headache and lethargy progressing rapidly to stupor and only after recovery from this serious position can language be evaluated. A dense total hemiplegia with variable degrees of sensory loss is a prominent finding.

The original language-finding is a true mutism (often during a period of decreased alertness); with return of verbalization marked hypophonia, dysarthria and decreased verbal agility are notable. The language output appears nonfluent in that it is sparse, dysarthric and has short phrase length. Effort and dysprosody, however, are not prominent. Verbalization is rare, usually follows external prompting and often incorporates some of the examiner's statement (but not to the degree called echolalia); just as frequently, the examiner's words are paraphrased. When encouraged to verbalize, the patient's output is severely contaminated by paraphasias, both literal and verbal. In contrast, comprehension of spoken language is relatively intact and repetition is remarkably accurate, up to a somewhat depressed span level. Confrontation-naming may be below normal but is far better than that seen in thalamic aphasia. Reading ability is disturbed but not completely lost and some words can be written by the left hand. Both striatal aphasia and thalamic aphasia are characterized by paraphasic conversational output in sharp contrast to the nonparaphasic repetition. They differ sharply, however, in the quantity and ease of the output; one resembles a nonfluent, anterior aphasia, the other a fluent posterior type. Striatal aphasia can be said to resemble the transcortical motor aphasia syndrome but the frequency of paraphasic errors during spontaneous conversation separates it from TCM and the other nonfluent aphasias.

Like thalamic aphasia, striatal aphasia tends to clear, although possibly not so completely. These patients often retain a dense right hemiplegia and a noticeable disturbance in the smoothness of verbal output. Whether the few personally observed cases which provided the descriptions given here will be replicated as additional cases are evaluated remains open. The CAT scan does allow demonstration of striatal hemorrhage in patients with aphasia and improved medical competence keeps more of these patients alive. Eventually a solid symptom picture should become available.

Three aphasic syndromes, each the result of hemorrhage into tissues deep in the dominant cerebral hemisphere, have been described. Obviously, considerable overlap both in the symptomatology and in the location of pathology must exist between the three syndromes. It should be equally obvious that all or part of any of these syndromes may occur in combination with language area cortical damage producing complex clusters of language symptoms. Recognition of the clinical picture produced by subcortical destruction may alleviate some of the confusion of mixed aphasia cases and offer valuable clinical and prognostic information.

APHASIA FROM WHITE MATTER LESIONS

One reason that aphasia has long been considered a strictly cortical abnormality by so many neurologists was the virtual absence of aphasia in CNS disorders that featured significant white matter pathology. The most striking example is multiple sclerosis (MS), a common neurologic disorder in which demyelination destroys much white matter but rarely involves the cortex primarily. While aphasia has been reported in sporadic cases of MS, it is notably uncommon (Almos-Lau, Ginsberg, Geller, 1977). Estimates of the frequency of aphasia in multiple sclerosis range from absolute zero (Kurtzke, 1970) to very rare (Muller, 1949). In contrast, speech disturbances are common, although not universal in MS. A study of speech quality in over one hundred individuals with a clinical diagnosis of multiple sclerosis at the Mayo Clinic showed slightly fewer than 50 percent with significant speech inadequacy (Darley, Aronson and Brown, 1975). Five major classes of speech abnormality are described in MS: 1) nasal voice, 2) weak phonation, 3) variability of pitch, 4) slow rate and 5) intellectual deterioration (Farmakides and Boone, 1960). The scanning speech emphasized by Charcot (1877) and widely taught as one of the diagnostic characteristics of MS is decidedly uncommon, seen only in the late stages of a few severe cases.

When aphasia is present in multiple sclerosis, one of two clinical pictures is typically seen. One rare type starts acutely with prominent motor language disturbance and right hemiplegia, is usually transient and resembles an acute vascular accident until later exacerbations point to the correct diagnosis (Adams and Victor, 1977). The second is an anomia occurring in the presence of progressive dementia including amnesia. In the former and many of the latter cases severe speech abnormality obscures the picture of aphasia. Whether the aphasia occasionally seen in MS actually results from subcortical (white matter) pathology remains unsettled. In the rare acute aphasia cases the possibility of cortical involvement by the placques or surrounding inflammation must be considered. In the chronic cases, the dementing process is so advanced that the language disability appears to be a minor accompaniment. Thus, aphasia is not only rare in multiple sclerosis, it can be earnestly questioned whether it ever occurs on the basis of pure white matter destruction.

Another subcortical white matter disorder, progressive multifocal leukoencephalopathy, has been reported as a cause of aphasia. One recent case (Buchwald, 1978) originally complained of only two symptoms, headache and severe anomia. The anomia was manifested by emptiness in conversational speech, distinct confrontation-naming failure and occasional verbal paraphasic substitutions. Repetition and comprehension were only mildly abnormal. The course was one of rapid deterioration, the patient sank into stupor and went on to an early demise. Data from CAT scans and the postmortem examination suggested (but did not prove) that the original lesion, the one underlying the anomia, involved white matter deep in the posterior temporal lobe on the left. It can be anticipated that additional cases of aphasia from white matter pathology will appear, particularly with the CAT scan's ability to demonstrate subcortical lesions. It remains striking, nonetheless, that aphasia is so rarely present in purely white matter disorders when involvement of the cortex is so regularly implicated.

10

Nonlocalizing Aphasic Syndromes

With some exceptions, the syndromes described so far have offered fairly replicable correlations between the clinical picture and a specific anatomic localization of pathology. Two major aphasic syndromes, however, do not offer such predictable localizations. One of these, anomic aphasia, is often believed to offer definitive localizing value but is readily and frequently misinterpreted. On the other hand, the second, global aphasia, is widely thought to be nonlocalizing when in actuality it often offers useful localizing information. These two "nonlocalizing" syndromes deserve careful consideration and will be discussed separately.

ANOMIC APHASIA

The disturbance we will call anomic aphasia is known by many other names including amnestic aphasia, amnesic aphasia and nominal aphasia. For many clinicians, anomic aphasia is the equivalent of anomia and thus represents any word-finding difficulty. This is not true, but as so few differentiating features separate anomic aphasia from anomia, this problem demands initial consideration.

Word-finding difficulty (anomia) is not only ubiquitous to aphasia but occurs in many nonaphasic disorders. The presence of anomia by itself fails to indicate an aphasic condition. Instead, word-finding difficulty presents a major problem in diagnostic differentiation. For instance:

1) Anomia is probably the most common finding in aphasia (although agraphia may be just as frequent); it is dangerous to consider a diagnosis of aphasia in a patient without anomia. For some investigators (Brown, 1972) anomia is the key disturbance in aphasia and underlies all the other disorders.

2) Anomia may be the only residual following recovery from aphasia (of any kind) and most recovered aphasics volunteer that they still suffer difficulty in word-finding to some degree.

3) Anomia is present, usually conspicuously so, in most varieties of dementia and is a diagnostic feature of the Alzheimer syndrome.

4) Word-finding defect is common in nonfocal brain disease such as increased intracranial pressure, subarachnoid hemorrhage, encephalitis, concussion, toxic-metabolic encephalopathy and many others.

5) Word-finding defects are a significant feature of the syndrome called

"nonaphasic misnaming" (Weinstein and Kahn, 1955; Weinstein and Keller, 1973), and on rare occasions in hysterical language difficulties (Geschwind, 1967b).

6) Anomia can take different appearances in a variety of aphasic syndromes. In particular, a word-production type of anomia is present in the anterior aphasias including Broca aphasia, transcortical motor aphasia and conduction aphasia. Either a word-selection anomia or a full blown semantic anomia or some combination occurs in posterior disorders such as Wernicke aphasia and the angular gyrus syndrome while category specific (color naming), modality specific (auditory agnosia) and callosal disconnection types of anomia occur following separation of primary sensory areas from the language area (Benson, 1979). Chapters 7–11, 13, 15 and 16 all contain descriptions of disorders in which some variety of word-finding deficit is prominent.

The present section will be restricted to the aphasic disorder in which word-finding defect is the only or the most conspicuous major component. This "pure" anomia can be called anomic aphasia and, when truly pure, is restricted to the word-selection type of anomia. Often, however, individual cases with semantic anomia are included if the word-finding defect outshadows the comprehension problem to a considerable degree. Chapter 15 offers further delineation of the types of anomia and Table 10-1 indicates the major diagnostic features of anomic aphasia.

Table 10-1. BASIC LANGUAGE CHARACTERISTICS
OF ANOMIC APHASIA

Conversational speech	Fluent, empty
Comprehension of spoken language	Normal to mild defect
Repetition of spoken language	Good
Confrontation-naming	Defective
Reading: Aloud	Good or defective
Comprehension	Good or defective
Writing	Good or defective

Despite its widespread recognition and apparently standard features, anomic aphasia has tremendous variations. The spontaneous speech may be striking and often diagnostic. While produced easily and fluently there is an emptiness, a lack of substantive words with the substitution of many nonspecific words that often fail to communicate the idea satisfactorily. Sentence structure is preserved except for word-finding pauses. Nouns, particularly proper names, are most involved but verbs and adjectives may also be affected. Replacement of specific words by generalizations, words or phrases of less exact meaning (thing, it, them, etc.) is common. The fluent output containing many indefinite words and few substantives produces a characteristic rambling and vague output called *empty speech*. Attempts may be made to substitute for the unavailable words, occasionally leading to semantic paraphasia. More often, excessive pauses typify the anomic output. An attempt may be made to substitute a description for an unavailable word. If the description demands a substantive word which cannot be produced another description may be tried. This rapidly produces a circuitous and unwieldy output called *circumlocution*. The characteristic features of anomic verbal output are readily noted.

Comprehension of spoken language may be fully normal in anomic aphasia. Not always is this true, however, and a fairly significant degree of comprehension disturbance may be present. Inasmuch as repetition is good (usually excellent) in anomic aphasia, a resemblance can be noted between anomic aphasia with comprehension disturbance and transcortical sensory aphasia with comparatively mild comprehension disturbance. In fact, anomic aphasia and transcortical sensory aphasia can be considered on a continuum with the differentiating factor being the degree of comprehension disturbance. The classic anomic aphasia, as already noted, should have comparatively good language comprehension.

Naming, of course, is disturbed. The degree varies widely, however, from case to case. Some show a barely discernible disturbance on confrontation-naming, whie in others confrontation-naming is severely disturbed. The patient with anomic aphasia, unable to name an object, usually does not benefit from prompting. In fact, patients with severe anomia often refuse to accept the correct names. Thus, if an object like a comb is presented not only will the name of the object be missing but when the object name is given by the examiner, the patient may state "you may call it a comb, but that's not the word I would use." There are significant differences between various types of word-finding problems. Chapter 15 will delineate some of these differences with suggested anatomical correlations. The ability to generate word lists, to name from a description and to name through modalities other than visual stimulation are usually affected, often to a significant degree, in anomic aphasia.

Reading and writing may be entirely normal but not infrequently there is abnormality of both. There is a fairly common syndrome in clinical practice in which the only aphasic disturbance is a serious anomia, accompanied by a complete alexia and agraphia (see Ch. 11). This syndrome (anomic aphasia, alexia and agraphia) plus the Gerstmann syndrome (see Ch. 16) almost invariably indicates significant structural damage to the dominant hemisphere angular gyrus.

As could be anticipated, the neighborhood neurologic signs are also variable. Often there are absolutely no associated neurologic signs at all. Hemiparesis, or even hemiplegia, hemisensory defect, visual field defect and many other disturbances may occur, however. In fact, because of the many types and locations of pathology capable of producing word-finding problems, either hemisphere may be involved. Thus, the patient with a mild anomia and severe hemiplegia may have pathology located deep in the dominant hemisphere or anywhere in the nondominant hemisphere. On the other hand, a severe word-finding defect but no neighborhood findings ("pure" anomic aphasia) suggests dominant posterior temporal defect.

Localization of the site of the lesion underlying anomia is possible through any of the popular techniques, but as the prior discussion suggested the potential sites are scattered. In some situations the actual size of the lesion may be too small for definitive demonstration by any contemporary techniques. On the other hand, the word-finding problem may represent a mere remnant of the original aphasia and does not reflect the size or site of lesion demonstrated. No large localizing study purports to demonstrate a definitive site for anomic aphasia.

The course of anomia is entirely dependent on the site and type of pathology. Anomia is often the lone residual of more severe aphasic disturbances. Patients with Broca aphasia, conduction aphasia, etc. can improve so that the only complaint is in word-finding. Most patients who have sustained a demonstrable aphasia, no matter how full the recovery, describe some degree of word-finding defect. Sometimes the anomia is too slight for notice by the casual observer but remains bothersome to the patient. Anomia remains the complaint of many well-recovered aphasics.

The etiology of anomia and anomic aphasia is notably variable. Almost any pathological process that can cause structural change in the brain can produce anomic aphasia. This includes cerebral vascular disease, tumor, trauma, abscess, encephalitis and degenerative disease. More than the other problems of language, pathology involving the cerebral tissue, particularly the cortex, of either hemisphere can produce a significant anomia.

As already noted, the neuroanatomic sites reported for anomic aphasia are widely variable. In a study by Gloning, Gloning and Hoff (1963), the location of pathology in patients with various aphasic syndromes including anomic aphasia was reported. Approximately 60 percent of patients with anomic aphasia had dominant hemisphere parietal-temporal junction locus for pathology; the other 40 percent, however, ranged over a wide territory. It is well-recognized that brain tumors distant from the dominant hemisphere language area can and do produce anomia. Even right hemisphere pathology is capable of producing word-finding problems. Thus, while a majority of patients with "pure" anomia will probably have dominant hemisphere parietal-temporal involvement, even this cannot be accepted as an absolute. It can be stated that anomic aphasia cannot be localized, although appropriate neighborhood neurological findings may help locate the pathology in some cases of anomia.

GLOBAL APHASIA

A disorder has long been recognized and frequently recorded in which all major language functions are seriously involved and is usually called total or global aphasia.

The clinical features are readily outlined as all major language functions including verbal output, comprehension, repetition, naming, reading and writing are severely disturbed. Despite this, considerable variation exists in the syndrome and each component will be discussed separately.

The verbal output in global aphasia is always limited although rarely to a state of true mutism. There is usually some ability to phonate and inflect and, with practice, even a single syllable output can be inflected sufficiently to present a language-like response. More often some ability to produce words is maintained. The words may be limited to expletives or a simple statement. It has long been suggested that when a single short phrase is constantly reiterated, no matter what the situation, the statement represents a phrase the patient was saying just prior to being struck down by the causative pathology. It is an attractive theory that remains unproved. Some patients inflect a single phoneme with enough skill to produce communication. Patients whose total verbal output is limited to strings of a single syllable such as "zu-zu-zu" or "tan-tan-tan" are not infrequent in clinical practice. In general, global aphasics produce few phonemes; the disorder has been called *phonemic disintegration* by Alajouanine (1956). Series speech is usually seriously limited but there are exceptions; some patients who cannot spontaneously utilize words will, with prompting, produce the beginning of a series such as counting, nursery rhymes, etc. The completion phenomenon is not seen.

Comprehension is frequently reported to be better than verbal output in global aphasia. Three reasons can be suggested. First, while true global aphasia includes a total loss of comprehension, lesser degrees of disability may exist so that some patients deserving the appelation, global aphasia, retain some ability to comprehend. Second, most global aphasics develop considerable skill at interpreting nonlanguage communication. They become remarkably alert to gestures, to vocal inflections and intonations and to nuances in facial and body postures. Many global aphasics become so sensitive to nonverbal communication that they fool family members and even trained examiners into believing that they comprehend much of what is being said. Most aphasiologists have experienced a family member reporting that an aphasic "understands everything I say" when testing reveals a total inability to interpret language. Finally, current insurance practices provide recompense for aphasia therapy but exclude global aphasia (because it is considered irreversible) and a statement that the patient has retained some comprehension allows financial support for a trial of language therapy. Thus, while there may be some ability to comprehend in some global aphasics, the amount reported is frequently exaggerated.

The patient with global aphasia does not repeat. If repetition is successfully performed, then one of the transcortical aphasic syndromes is present. Similarly, naming is severely, usually totally, disturbed as are reading and writing. In fact, as stated, the patient with global aphasia has severe deficits in all aspects of language.

Attempts have been made to define global aphasia on a quantitative basis from several aphasia batteries. The PICA (Porch, 1967) is particularly adept at this diagnostic task. In essence anyone who scores less than 6.0 on the PICA can be considered to have a severe global aphasia. It is also possible to set parameters on the BDAE which demarcate global aphasia. A patient who scores more than 1.5 standard deviations below normal on each major language subtest is considered to have global aphasia (Goodglass and Kaplan, 1972). Tests for global aphasia, however, both standardized batteries and clinical evaluations, often fail to demonstrate significant variations. As already noted, global aphasia does not represent a single, consistent syndrome and additional studies directed toward the variation in findings will further define this group and possibly indicate separate syndromes.

The neighborhood neurologic signs most often indicate severe brain damage. These usually include hemiplegia (or bilateral hemiplegia), sensory loss, visual field loss and often an attention disturbance. The disturbance almost invariably involves the right side of the body but indication of bilateral pathology is common. Surprisingly, a fully global aphasia may be present in a patient with only minimal basic neurologic deficit. A number of explanations have been formulated for this unexpected discrepancy, but to date all remain unproved.

Localization procedures including EEG, radioisotope scanning, CAT scanning, surgical excision and autopsy consistently report large lesions involving much of the language area of the dominant hemisphere in cases of global aphasia.

The course in global aphasia is more variable than usually recorded. Many patients who present with global aphasia at the onset rapidly change to one of the other standard aphasic syndromes. If the patient fails to improve and a severe global aphasia remains unaltered for a prolonged period, several interpretations can be suggested. Smith (1972) suggests that the lack of improvement indicates bilateral brain damage but others suggest that consistent global aphasia can result from severe unilateral, dominant hemisphere damage. Those who do not make a rapid recovery from global aphasia soon after onset have a poor prognosis; many remain severely or completely language deficient. Life expectancy is not necessarily affected by the disorder and many unfortunates live for years with severe global aphasia. It has long been accepted that chronic global aphasia does not respond to aphasia therapy, but recent innovations in therapy technique may alter this grim picture (see Ch. 18).

The etiologic factors underlying global aphasia include almost anything capable of severely damaging the left hemisphere. Cerebral vascular accident is probably most common but tumor, trauma, infection, gunshot wound, surgical intervention and others can all lead to severe global aphasia.

Anatomically, global aphasia is most often the product of pathology involving the dominant hemisphere middle cerebral artery territory. The pathology may be quite extensive, involving much of the hemisphere (or as noted above, both hemispheres) but global aphasia can occur after considerably less pathology. One suggested source of global aphasia with comparatively minimal neighborhood neurologic findings is an infarct along the sylvian lips, involving the posterior-inferior frontal region, the posterior-superior temporal region and other immediate perisylvian tissues but not involving motor association cortex, sensory association cortex or the visual pathways. While global aphasia appears to have some localizing value, there is so much variation within the syndrome that it is not wise to suggest specific localization on the basis of the language findings of global aphasia alone.

11

Alexia

Alexia refers to a disturbance in reading and may be defined simply as the loss or impairment of the ability to read caused by brain damage, equivalent to the definition of aphasia except for the restriction to written or printed language. Again, one key consideration in the definition is the concept of loss. Alexia is an acquired disorder. To emphasize this point many contemporary students of the topic distinguish alexia from dyslexia but the distinction is semantically artificial and not universally accepted. With this usage, however, the term *alexia* is limited to situations in which the ability to read was present and became lost after brain damage, whereas *dyslexia* refers to a developmental abnormality in which the individual is unable to learn to read. Dyslexia is thus defined as an inherent inability to learn to comprehend written or printed words and is a very different disorder. The difference goes well beyond a mere matter of semantics; the clinical findings and the treatment of the two disorders are totally different. Another crucial consideration is that the function of reading in the definition of alexia refers strictly to the comprehension of written material. The ability to read out loud is often a separate function: loss of the ability to read aloud without disturbance of the ability to comprehend written language should not be called alexia. On the other hand, a person who can read aloud but fails to comprehend the material should be called alexic.

Several other terms from the alexia lexicon deserve mention. *Literal alexia* refers to a comparative inability to read (name) individual letters of the alphabet and in the older terminology was called *letter-blindness*. *Verbal alexia* refers to an inability to read words (aloud and for comprehension) in the face of comparative retention of letter recognition and has been called *word-blindness*.

HISTORICAL BACKGROUND

Alexia has been recognized for centuries but only in the 20th century has literacy become sufficiently widespread for alexia to be a significant medical problem. While there are reports of alexia preceding the time of Christ and many recorded incidents of alexia prior to the time of Broca (Benton, 1964), even the surge in language study of the 19th century produced only limited interest in alexia. The major impetus to the understanding of alexia dates from two case reports published by Dejerine in 1891 and 1892. In the 1891 paper Dejerine described an individual who suffered a cerebral vascular accident following which he could no longer read. The patient originally had a mild right-sided weakness, some degree of right-sided visual field defect and mild difficulty in other language functions. In addition to the alexia the patient totally lost the ability to write except for his signature. The aphasia cleared almost completely but the alexia and agraphia remained severe until death several years later. At postmortem the brain had an old, scarred infarct involving three quarters of the cortex of the angular gyrus and extending deep to the lateral ventricle in the left parietal lobe. Pathological destruction of most of the dominant angular gyrus had produced an acquired illiteracy.

In a separate report published a year later, Dejerine described a patient who suddenly lost the ability to read but had no other language disturbance. The only neurologic finding of significance was a right homonymous hemianopsia. Unlike the original patient, this individual, while unable to read except for some individual letters, could write adequately. A second major cerebral vascular accident a number of years later led to death 10 days later and postmortem examination revealed two clearly different infarcts. One was a large softening involving the dominant hemisphere angular gyrus that was obviously of recent origin. The second was an old, scarred infarction that involved the medial and inferior aspects of the left occipital lobe and the splenium of the corpus callosum. Dejerine conjectured that the original infarct had destroyed the visual pathways leading to the visual cortex of the dominant hemisphere occipital area causing the right visual field defect, and that the callosal lesion had separated the intact right hemisphere visual area from the equally intact left hemisphere language area. Thus the patient suffered no language defect except the inability to interpret written language symbols.

Table 11-1. TERMINOLOGY OF THE ALEXIAS

Parietal-Temporal alexia	Occipital alexia	Frontal alexia
Alexia with agraphia	Alexia without agraphia	
Central alexia	Posterior alexia	Anterior alexia
Associative alexia	Sensory alexia	Motor alexia
Aphasic alexia	Agnosic alexia	
Cortical alexia	Optic alexia	
Word and letter blindness	"Pure" word blindness	"Pure" letter blindness
Total alexia	Verbal alexia	Literal alexia
Secondary alexia	Primary alexia	Tertiary alexia
Perceptive alexia	Receptive alexia	Expressive alexia
Semantic alexia		Syntactic alexia

Dejerine's reports excited many investigators and in the next few years a number of case reports of alexia were published supporting the clinical and neuropathological pattern described by Dejerine (Wylie, 1894; Bastian, 1898; Hinshelwood, 1900). From this time two varieties of alexia have traditionally been accepted, *alexia with agraphia* indicating a dominant parietal lobe lesion and *alexia without agraphia* with pathology damaging the dominant occipital lobe and the splenium of the corpus callosum. It has always been apparent, however, that many patients with significant alexia did not have pathology in either of these sites. Recently a third, clinically distinct variety of alexia associated with pathology in the frontal language areas has been demonstrated (Benson, 1977). The following discussion will focus on these three varieties of alexia and outline a few other disturbances easily mistaken for alexia. Historically, many different terms have been used to delineate the varieties of alexia, producing a fertile field for confusion (see Table 11-1). For this report, the three major syndromes will be discussed under the suggested neuroanatomical loci of pathology, an arbitrary and artificial division which has as much or as little specificity as any of the other divisions.

PARIETAL-TEMPORAL ALEXIA

The syndrome most often called alexia *with* agraphia has been described many times in the literature. The symptom picture is striking and comparatively precise but the neighborhood findings vary considerably, dependent upon the amount and the location of cerebral pathology.

The major features are, of course, the disturbances of reading and writing, the alexia and agraphia. The loss of these abilities may be total but often occurs in degrees of incompleteness. Not only is the ability to read both letters and words impaired, but as a rule there is equal difficulty in comprehension of numbers and musical notation. The ability to read out loud and the ability to comprehend written language are both disturbed. Cues are of little help. Thus, tracing the letter with the finger does not aid in identification and the patient with a parietal-temporal alexia cannot decipher a word when it is spelled aloud for him. In fact the patient often volunteers that he cannot understand a word spelled aloud because he cannot read.

The writing disturbance in parietal-temporal alexia is usually of equal severity. While the patient may produce some real letters and combinations of letters which resemble words, most of the letter combinations fail to show specific meaning. The ability to copy written and printed words is far better than the ability to produce them on command. Often, however, the patient will be unable to transpose cursive to printed form or vice versa. The patient with parietal-temporal alexia can be considered illiterate for written and printed language symbols; it is an acquired illiteracy.

Significant neurologic and neurobehavioral findings may or may not be present. Right hemiparesis is frequently seen early but most often disappears in a short time. Right-sided sensory loss is more common and tends to remain as a permanent difficulty. Either a right homonymous hemianopsia or a right superior quadrantanopsia may be present, depending on involvement of the visual pathways, but many cases without visual field defect have been recorded. A variety of aphasic findings may be present; these can include paraphasic verbal output, defective comprehension of spoken language, inability to repeat and/or anomia; in rare instances all signs of aphasia may be absent, however. The Gerstmann syndrome (see Ch. 16) is often present as are constructional disturbances and deterioration of intellectual capacity. None of the above findings are consistently present and none are necessary for the diagnosis. Alexia with agraphia can be seen completely separate from any neighborhood findings, particularly in the chronic state, although this is exceptional.

Localization of the site of pathology is frequently determined by the accompanying neurologic defects and may be confirmed by CAT and isotope brain scans, surgical exploration and autopsy examinations. Trauma to the brain with focal skull defects has also been used to localize the pathology of parietal-temporal alexia.

The course of parietal-temporal alexia is remarkably variable, dependent on the underlying etiology and the size of the lesion. Rapid recovery of some or all reading skills is not uncommon. More often there is a partial recovery, permitting only limited reading comprehension, and not infrequently the acquired illiteracy remains unaltered from the day of inception. Obviously, the recovery is influenced by the premorbid literacy level and the importance of reading in the lifestyle of the patient. Many patients have never been regular readers and demonstrate little concern over their acquired illiteracy. Unfortunately, some patients who most strongly desire resumption of literacy maintain their alexia and agraphia indefinitely.

A variety of disease processes are capable of producing parietal-temporal alexia. Most common is cerebral vascular disease, particularly occlusion of the angular branch of the middle cerebral artery. Not infrequently the etiology is a parietal arterial-venous malformation or an infiltrating glioma. Trauma, gunshot wound, abscess and metastatic tumor are less frequent as sources of the syndrome. Despite the primary location of pathology in a portion of the vascular borderzone, alexia with agraphia is not commonly reported as the primary syndrome after great vessel occlusion; if present, the alexic syndrome is obscured by additional language defects and becomes part of a larger symptom complex (often transcortical sensory aphasia).

The presence of alexia with agraphia was originally reported following dominant hemisphere angular gyrus damage. Multiple subsequent reports have supported this localization (Benson and Geschwind, 1969). The pathology often involves surrounding cerebral areas, particularly the immediately adjacent temporal lobe structures and, as already noted, may be accompanied by a wide variety of findings. The body of recorded cases of alexia with agraphia showing pathology in the parietal-temporal junction area is large with only rare reports of other sites involved in cases of this syndrome.

One association of findings (syndrome) frequently noted in clinical practice includes alexia with agraphia, the Gerstmann syndrome and anomia. This cluster has been called the angular gyrus syndrome and almost invariably indicates a dominant hemisphere inferior parietal location of the causative pathology.

OCCIPITAL ALEXIA

The syndrome often called alexia *without* agraphia is spectacular but not common. As Table 11-1 indicates, the syndrome has been called many different names, the most popular of which are pure alexia, pure word blindness, agnosic alexia, occipital alexia, optic aphasia and, of course, alexia without agraphia. Occipital alexia is a comparatively specific syndrome, and because of the dramatic findings it tends to be recognized by clinicians. The definitive findings are a serious inability to read contrasted with an almost uncanny preservation of writing ability. The patient with "pure" alexia actually finds himself unable to read what he has just finished writing. Most patients with occipital alexia can understand some common written words such as the name of their city and state, their own name, "USA" and other commonly used language symbols, but they will fail to read many others. Most of these patients eventually regain the ability to read many or all individual letters and can read them aloud. At first this process is performed slowly and insecurely but if the letters of a word are read aloud, the patient can often put them together so that the word can be deciphered. This patient has a verbal alexia but not a literal alexia. Obviously, the process of reading individual letters aloud and then recognizing the spelled word is slow and open to error, particularly on longer words dependent upon a suffix for exact meaning (e.g. they read refrigerator for refrigeration, medical for medicine, etc.). When a word is spelled out loud by the examiner, the patient with occipital alexia will immediately recognize the word, a sharp contrast to the situation in parietal-temporal alexia where this task is totally failed. Recognition of spelled words becomes an important differentiating test for these two varieties of alexia. With continued improvement, the "reading" becomes speedier; it no longer is necessary to spell out loud but the "reading" is still accomplished by identifying individual letters and putting them together to form words. The patient with occipital alexia can also recognize individual letters when they are drawn in the palm or palpated from embossed blocks, and can decipher words presented in this manner at about the same speed as normal control subjects. Thus, the patient with occipital alexia has not lost the power to read; rather, it appears that visual stimuli have only limited access to the language area.

Neurologic and neurobehavioral findings in occipital alexia are also striking and sufficiently consistent to be aids in diagnosis. As already noted, patients with occipital alexia usually write without difficulty. They can write full personal letters or long paragraphs of description, only to find at the end of the task that they can neither read nor remember what they have just written. Some patients with occipital alexia suffer minor writing difficulties, particularly a tendency to slant their writing upwards (Martin, 1954) and a tendency for the writing to deteriorate over the years (Adler, 1950), possibly based on the long absence of visual monitoring. Patients with occipital alexia have greater difficulty copying written material than in producing words to dictation, again a sharp contrast to the performance of patients with a parietal-temporal alexia. If asked to spell words out loud, patients with occipital alexia perform excellently, which is yet another differentiating feature of this disorder.

Right homonymous hemianopsia is present in most cases of occipital alexia but a number of individual cases of occipital alexia have been described in which there was no hemianopsia (Ajax, 1967; Goldstein, Joynt and Goldblatt, 1971). Most cases without hemianopsia have been due to tumor, either a meningioma compressing the medial occipital region or a glioma infiltrating this region. In contrast, the majority of reported cases of occipital alexia have been secondary to vascular disease and significant unilateral visual field defect has been present in most.

While most language functions are normal or near normal, many patients with occipital alexia have great difficulty naming colors. Also, if the process is reversed with the patient asked to point to a color named by the examiner, the problem is just as severe. These patients have no difficulty using color names in conversation or in auditory comprehension (i.e. what is the color of a banana?) and they can sort colors easily and accurately. Only in the visual-verbal association process of naming a color or pointing to a named color do they fail. This is a two-way defect and can be considered a true agnosia for colors (Geschwind and Fusillo, 1966). Not all patients with occipital alexia have color-naming disturbance, but in one large series (Gloning, Gloning and Hoff, 1963) "color-naming disturbance" was present in over 70 percent of the cases of "pure" alexia.

Other neighborhood findings occur with less consistency. Many individuals with occipital alexia have a mild degree of anomia, less than the color-naming disturbance but still appreciable. Some have difficulty in number-reading and others suffer a true acalculia. Musical notation-reading is lost in some, but not in others. The most significant neighborhood findings, however, are negative; there is an absence of paralysis, sensory deficit or any other basic neurologic defect except for the right homonymous hemianopsia and there is no disturbance in language function (aphasia).

Because of the rather unusual and separated neuroanatomical locus of pathology underlying occipital alexia, many techniques successfully demonstrate the site of the lesion. A number of autopsied cases have been reported (Benson and Geschwind, 1969) and other successful localizing techniques including the CAT scan, the isotope brain scan, EEGs and even angiography have demonstrated occlusion of the dominant hemisphere posterior cerebral artery.

The course of occipital alexia varies but a slow, persistent improvement is common and reading ability eventually improves to a level of usefulness. Treatment, including use of elementary reading materials and large print newspapers and books, plus a considerable amount of encouragement, are often rewarded by obvious improvement. The patient's reading ability, however, rarely returns to normal or even to a level of reading for pleasure.

Both the pathology and the site of lesion are remarkably consistent in occipital alexia. The anatomical defect described by Dejerine can be demonstrated in most cases. Usually the defect results from a cerebral vascular accident (occlusion of the left posterior cerebral artery) but the syndrome has also been

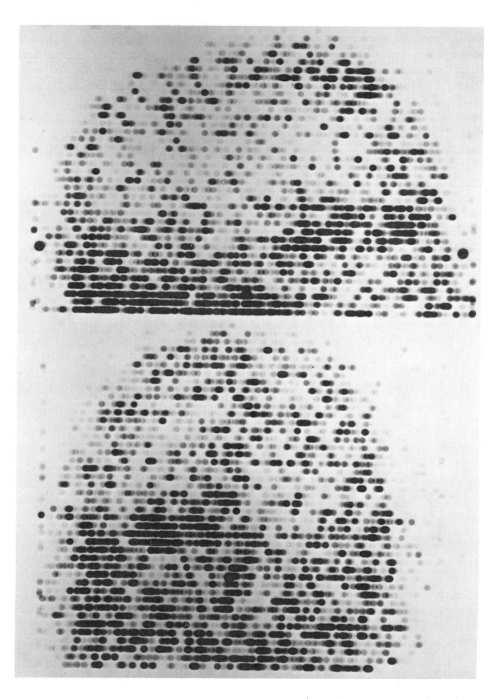

Figure 11-1. *Radioisotope scan (left lateral and PA) showing increased uptake in the territory of the left posterior cerebral artery. The patient had the features of posterior alexia (alexia without agraphia).*

described with tumors and AV malformation. The cerebral destruction is centered in the medial, inferior occipital region, usually affecting the fusiform and lingual gyri and involving the posterior segment of the geniculo-calcarine pathway. In addition, pathological involvement of the splenium of the corpus callosum is present in most cases. In the few cases of occipital alexia in which splenial pathology was not reported, either pathology involving the deep white matter immediately adjacent to the splenium has been reported, or the pathologist has failed to report (and presumably to investigate) the condition of the splenium.

As a separate but closely related entity, Greenblatt (1976) has suggested an entity that he called *subangular alexia*. In the case that he reported the patient had alexia without either agraphia or hemianopsia. In similar cases quoted from the literature by Greenblatt, alexia and aphasia were present but hemianopsia was not. The structural pathology in these cases involved the white matter deep in the dominant parietal cortex, undercutting the angular gyrus. The presence of alexia without agraphia suggested that the "subangular" lesion acted to disconnect the intact dominant hemisphere angular gyrus from visual stimuli arising from both the right and left hemispheres but did not otherwise interfere with angular gyrus function. Subangular alexia, then, can be considered a separate syndrome, midway between parietal-temporal alexia and occipital alexia, but clinically most closely related to the latter. A detailed discussion of variations in the symptom picture between that of parietal-temporal alexia and occipital alexia, coupled with posited underlying neuroanatomical variations, has been presented recently by Greenblatt (1977).

FRONTAL ALEXIA

The third variety of alexia to be discussed has a long and controversial history. For many years it has been noted that many patients with Broca aphasia lose the ability to read. Just how a frontal alexia could be explained, using the prevalent theories of language, was never settled. In fact, Freud (1891) used the combination of Broca aphasia and alexia as a major argument to disprove the localization theories of language prevalent in the 1890's. For many of the cases of anterior aphasia with alexia reported in the last century, the inability to read could merely represent a poor premorbid reading ability. With the spread of literacy in the 20th century, this explanation can no longer be accepted. Alexia is frequently present in individuals with aphasia caused by frontal pathology. In a review of 61 cases of Broca aphasia evaluated at the Boston Veterans Administration Hospital, 51 showed a significant degree of alexia (Benson, 1977).

A number of features of frontal alexia are sufficiently distinctive to allow differentiation from the other two varieties of alexia (see Table 11-2). Most patients with frontal alexia do understand some written material; usually this is limited to individual words, characteristically nouns or action verbs. Sometimes, these patients can decipher a newspaper headline but will fail to com-

Table 11-2. DIFFERENTIATING FEATURES OF THE THREE ALEXIAS

	Parietal-Temporal	Occipital	Frontal
Written Language			
1) Reading	Total alexia	Primarily verbal alexia	Primarily literal alexia
2) Writing	Severe agraphia except for copy	No agraphia	Severe agraphia including copy
3) Letter-naming	Severe anomia for letters	Comparatively intact	Severe anomia for letters
4) Comprehension of spelled words	Failed	Good	Partial success
5) Spelling out loud	Failed	Good	Poor
Associated Findings			
1) Language	Fluent aphasia	Normal	Nonfluent aphasia
2) Motor	Mild paresis	Normal	Hemiplegia
3) Sensory	Hemisensory loss	Normal	Mild sensory loss
4) Visual field	May or may not have field defect	Right hemianopsia	Usually normal
5) Gerstmann syndrome	Frequent	Absent	Absent

prehend the sentences that make up the article. Most can read, both aloud and for comprehension, but only isolated words from a given sentence; the recognized words are almost exclusively substantives. If a word can be read aloud it will be understood and vice versa. If the meaning of a sentence depends upon only one or two substantive words, the patient may guess the meaning of the entire sentence. If, however, relational words such as adjectives, prepositional phrases and such are the determining language structures, the patient may completely misinterpret the sentence. Even as they prove that they understand some words, they insist that they cannot read and consistently avoid reading. In contrast to occipital alexia, these individuals can read some words but fail when asked to read (name) individual letters of the word. Patients with frontal alexia show a severe literal alexia and a lesser degree of verbal alexia (Benson, Brown and Tomlinson, 1971). The patient may recognize some words spelled aloud (most often substantive words) but fails to recognize most.

A severe writing disturbance is almost always present with frontal alexia. The writing, most often performed with the left hand, is crude and poorly formed and the spelling is faulty. While they can copy written language, they have much greater difficulty in this task than patients with the other two types of alexia. Even in copying, the production is badly formed and there is a tendency to omit letters.

The associated findings of frontal alexia are distinct and very helpful in confirming the diagnosis. In the first place, nonfluent aphasia, most frequently Broca aphasia, is usually present. Some studies (Hecaen and Albert, 1978) suggest that many patients with transcortical motor aphasia comprehend written material adequately. This is in contrast to the reading ability in Broca aphasia. While the verbal output of patients with frontal alexia is usually limited, comprehension of spoken language is comparatively good, much better than comprehension of written language. Right hemiplegia is usually present and a sizeable number will show some degree of sensory loss and visual field defect (Benson, 1977). Frontal alexia has a tendency to remain severe, often becoming the most disabling residual following a good recovery from Broca aphasia. On the other hand, some individuals with Broca aphasia show no alexia whatsoever and alexia cannot be considered a consistent feature of Broca aphasia. In summary, as Table 11-2 demonstrates, sufficient differentiating findings are present to clearly separate frontal alexia from the other two varieties.

Demonstration of the neuroanatomic locus of pathology in frontal alexia has been by the same means used to localize frontal aphasic lesions. Definitive autopsy studies (Nielsen, 1936) support clinical and laboratory techniques delineating the site of lesions in cases of frontal alexia.

The pathology in frontal alexia is located in the anterior portion of the dominant hemisphere, involving the posterior portion of the inferior frontal gyrus with extension into the subcortical tissues in the anterior insula. Whether a reading disturbance occurs with involvement of other sites in the frontal language area has not been validated. The underlying etiology of frontal alexia is the same as that causing Broca aphasia with cerebral vascular problems predominating.

Finally, it should be emphasized that the complaint of difficulty in reading claimed by these patients is quite real. While they can decipher some words, the degree of reading impairment is significant and deserves being classed as a true alexia. It is not, however, the full illiteracy of parietal-temporal alexia and differs from occipital alexia in many features. Table 11-2 outlines distinctive characteristics of both the reading and writing and the associated signs that help differentiate the three major varieties of alexia.

OTHER VARIETIES OF READING DISTURBANCE

Hemialexia

There are a few cases reported in the literature in which the splenium of the corpus callosum was purposely cut but no damage was incurred by occipital tissues in either hemisphere. In some, particularly those reported by Akelaitis (1941, 1943, 1944), no difficulty with reading was observed; other case reports (Trescher and Ford, 1937; Maspes, 1948; Gazzaniga and Sperry, 1967) in which the splenium of the corpus callosum was severed demonstrated loss of the ability to understand written material visualized in the left visual field (right hemisphere). Preserved ability to read material in the right visual field (left hemisphere) was present in each case, producing a condition that can be called *hemialexia*. Hemialexia is rare and appears, symptomatically, closely related to the syndrome of occipital alexia. Hemialexia has only been reported following neurosurgical severance of the posterior part of the corpus callosum, but at least in theory it could occur with other pathology involving the splenium only.

Aphasic Alexia

Alexia occurs as a feature of many aphasic syndromes and may be considered a part of the language disturbance in these. One, that associated with the anterior aphasias (Broca and transcortical motor aphasia), has been described separately as frontal alexia and need not be discussed further. Two of the posterior aphasia syndromes, Wernicke aphasia and transcortical sensory aphasia, are consistently associated with alexia. In transcortical sensory aphasia the causative pathology often involves the angular gyrus and the resulting alexia is similar or identical to the parietal-temporal variety of alexia already described. Many cases with the clinical features of Wernicke aphasia also have pathology that affects the angular gyrus (Wernicke's area of the temporal lobe and the angular gyrus of the parietal lobe are contiguous regions without a clear anatomical demarcation) and a similar correlation can be suggested. Not all cases of Wernicke aphasia have pathological involvement of the angular gyrus, however. Cases of Wernicke aphasia have been reported in which the patient was totally unable to comprehend written material but at postmortem showed no extension of pathology into the angular gyrus. Neilsen (1938) reported 16 such cases and conjectured, as had others before him, that as we master an auditory language thoroughly before attempting to understand a visual language, the visual language is learned by association with the overlearned auditory language. Thus, pathology involving auditory comprehension areas alone could interfere with the associations necessary for reading. Whether this explanation is accepted or not, it appears that temporal lobe pathology causing Wernicke aphasia but without any encroachment on the parietal lobe can produce an alexia which is similar if not identical to parietal-temporal alexia.

Varieties of Pseudoalexia

A number of disturbances of reading ability are recognized that resemble alexia but, following careful testing, fail to fit the definition. They have been called *pseudoalexia* (Benson and Geschwind, 1969).

The most common source of an "untrue" alexia stems from a partially performed evaluation, particularly when the ability to read out loud is the only reading function tested. Patients with severe speech problems (such as are seen in the anterior aphasias or subcortical movement disorders) may fail to read out loud and yet comprehend written material adequately. Exactly this finding is a common feature in conduction aphasia where the discrepancy between the ability to read out loud and the ability to comprehend written material can be an important differentiating finding (Benson et al, 1973). Loss of the ability to read out loud does not indicate alexia; only loss of the ability to comprehend written material can be called alexia.

Unilateral paralexia is another condition that is easily mistaken for alexia. In this condition a patient, most commonly following acute loss of one homonymous visual field, may fail to read (neglect) one side of a word or a sentence. Thus a patient with a right visual field defect may read the word "southeast" as "south," while the patient with an acute left visual field loss may read the same word as "east." At times the patient may substitute (confabulate) the portions of the word that falls in the blind field ("southern" for "southeast"). Patients with unilateral paralexia often have considerable difficulty comprehending written material and are easily thought to have alexia. That this is not a true alexia can be demonstrated by writing a word or sentence in a vertical line rather than the traditional horizontal fashion (Kinsbourne and Warrington, 1962). The patient with unilateral paralexia may misread the horizontally presented material but correctly read the same material presented vertically. The disturbance is a manifestation of unilateral inattention (see Ch. 16) and is not a true alexia.

Mental retardation and *developmental dyslexia* can both be misinterpreted and lead to an incorrect diagnosis of alexia. Many mentally retarded individuals never learn to read just as some otherwise normal individuals with developmental dyslexia never master the skill. If an individual with either of these problems suffers an acute cerebral lesion later in life, examination will demonstrate the inability to comprehend written material and can lead to a misdiagnosis of alexia. Only careful history-taking protects the clinician from this dilemma.

Finally there are a few recorded cases of *psychogenic pseudoalexia*. A claim to have lost the ability to read is rare as a psychogenic defense mechanism, and when seen it is usually part of a far more extensive pseudodementia picture. If the clinician is aware of the common characteristics and associated neurologic findings of the alexias there should be little problem in separating out this entity. Discovery of the underlying cause of a psychogenic pseudoalexia may pose a much harder problem, however.

Alexia in Oriental Languages

All discussion so far has concerned alexia in English or related Indo-European languages. There is good reason to suspect that acquired disturbances of written language may be considerably different in the Oriental languages, particularly those languages that utilize both ideographic and phonetic characters. The medical literature now contains considerable case material outlining this difference, particularly the recent works from Japan (Sasanuma and Fujimura, 1971; Yamadori, 1975), demonstrating differences between the alexia of Kana (phonetic, syllabic) and Kanji (nonphonetic, logographic or ideographic) written characters. While the number of cases reported to date is limited, patients with more posterior (parietal-occipital) dominant hemisphere lesions apparently sustain greater loss in Kanji while patients with more anterior (temporal-parietal) pathology have most difficulty with the Kana script. These findings correlate with the stronger visual aspects of the Kanji and the stronger auditory aspects of the Kana characters.

Reading with the Right Hemisphere

In the discussion of hemialexia it was suggested that, following section of the splenium of the corpus callosum, patients could read with the left hemisphere but not with the right. Clinical observations also indicate that most humans do not read well with their right hemisphere. Many patients with left hemisphere pathology develop and maintain a true alexia despite their normal right hemisphere. There are remarkably few recorded cases of alexia following right hemisphere pathology (Gloning et al, 1955) or of intact reading ability despite severe left hemisphere pathology producing aphasia. Clinical observations strongly imply that the ability to comprehend written language demands an intact dominant hemisphere in most adults and, conversely, the presence of alexia indicates dominant hemisphere pathology.

There is evidence, however, that the right hemisphere is capable of some comprehension of written language. Most of this evidence comes from the investigation of patients who have undergone section of the corpus callosum, for control of epilepsy. A limited ability to read (interpret written material) with their isolated right hemisphere has been demonstrated in some of these patients (Gazzaniga and Sperry, 1967; Bogen, 1969; Gazzaniga, 1970). The most striking examples followed presentation of written words tachistiscopically to the left visual field. The patient states that no word has been seen (the left hemisphere is doing the talking) but the left hand will reach out and pick up the object named in the written presentation. The results are consistent and clearly demonstrate that the right hemisphere of these patients has some ability to comprehend written material. There are some special features of these cases, however. In particular, all of the patients in these studies had serious seizure problems which dated from early childhood and the question can be asked whether they had ever achieved a normal lateralization of language function. With such strong clinical evidence suggesting that alexia improves even less than aphasia, it would appear that the ability of the right hemisphere to take over reading comprehension must be limited, at best.

There is one other bit of information, however, which suggests that the right hemisphere may be able to take over some reading tasks. A number of cases have been seen in which patients with severe left hemisphere language dysfunction, including severe parietal-temporal alexia, have, after a number of years, developed a limited ability to comprehend some parts of written language. Their reading has been limited to substantive, picturable words, most often words that are seen frequently. Thus a housewife may learn to recognize the words "milk" or "bread" because she sees the printed words so often in the context of the actual object. Some patients have been described in whom this type of reading has been carried even further; however, they make characteristic errors that are informative. Thus, such a patient might read "infant" as "baby," "automobile" as "car," etc. It has been suggested that in this condition the right hemisphere associates the written word with a visual image and can then name the visual image. If more than one name could be correct for the visualized image, the patient may choose the incorrect synonym. This phenomenon has been termed *paralexia* and is most often seen in individuals who have had a long course of temporal-parietal alexia.

In summary, alexia is not a single language dysfunction, but is rather a complex of distinctive disorders. As such, the careful study of alexia offers valuable neuroanatomical localizing information.

12

Agraphia

Agraphia may be defined simply as a loss or impairment of the ability to produce written language, caused by brain damage. There is nothing simple about agraphia, however. In fact, disturbances of written language have proved so complex that they have defied useful clinical correlation to date. One exception, a simple rule of thumb concerning agraphia, can be of considerable significance in the evaluation of aphasia. Almost without exception, every individual with aphasia will show at least some degree of agraphia and tests of writing capability can be used as a screening device for the presence of aphasia. Caution is necessary, however, as agraphia accompanies many disturbances other than aphasia. It would appear that writing is, at best, a tenuous accomplishment for most humans and that almost any brain abnormality can produce considerable disruption of writing skill.

Written language is a form of language and, as such, should mirror the complexities of language and language loss. The varieties of aphasia can be reflected by the varieties of agraphia but many other elements, unrelated to aphasia, are also of importance in writing. For instance, visual spatial abnormalities will have a considerable influence on writing. Written language is a rigidly exact, precise output produced in a specific spatial orientation; constructional skills are necessary to form meaningful language symbols (letters) and abnormality of visual spatial discrimination, of spatial orientation or of constructional skill will produce nonaphasic varieties of agraphia. Similarly, motor abnormality will cause serious problems in written language production. Ataxia, rigidity, spasticity, chorea and myoclonus involving the dominant limb cause major alterations in the quality of graphic output. Paralysis is a source of abnormal written language that is easily recognized and, as such, tends to be overemphasized. Many aphasics are paralyzed in the upper extremity favored for writing (usually the right), demanding that the task be attempted with the other (left) hand. Poor writing is frequently explained by noting that the patient must use the nonfavored hand, most often a false conception. Right-handed individuals forced to use the left hand because of right upper extremity injury rapidly produce an acceptable written language. The linguistic and motor quality of their writing is remarkably better than the agraphic output of the aphasic patient with right hemiparesis. Aphasic agraphia cannot be rationalized simply as a disturbed production based on use of the nonfavored extremity. Nonetheless, the disturbed motor competency of the nonpreferred hand also affects the quality of the written output in many aphasic patients.

With so many potential complexities clouding the features of written language, it is not surprising that agraphia has proved a difficult topic to analyze. While there have been attempts to utilize graphic evaluation for clinical purposes, using both anatomical and psychological correlations, none have proved consistently useful to date.

TESTING FOR AGRAPHIA

Although a simple outline to guide analysis of written production in aphasia was offered in Chapter 4, additional tests and interpretations are necessary for the present discussion.

Automatic writing skills should be tested carefully but may prove confusing unless interpreted critically. The signature is the most highly overlearned writing capability of any individual and a request to sign the name is often performed quite well by aphasic patients. If testing is discontinued at this point (not uncommon in clinical practice) the examiner may erroneously conclude that the patient has no agraphia. Many aphasic patients sign their name flawlessly but cannot write any other words or even letters on request. Other automatic writing such as address, home town, state, numbers, letters of the alphabet and days of the week are far less overlearned and many patients with aphasia will not be able to write them. Nonetheless, performance in automatic writing tasks tends to be far superior to other, less overlearned written functions. The value of testing the automatic writing skills is twofold. First, it helps establish a set (writing) for the more difficult requests that follow, and second, it demonstrates the best possible written production, particularly valuable for the patient forced to write with an unaccustomed limb because of hemiparesis.

The second step in testing agraphia is a request to copy words and sentences written by the examiner. Copying can be performed without comprehension of the linguistic content, although most normal individuals do analyze and comprehend as they copy. For instance, normal subjects can copy nonsense words or words in a foreign language that are not understood, and many patients with significant language comprehension defect can copy without difficulty. By itself, copying is not a sufficient test for agraphia, but it clearly demonstrates spatial disturbances which may affect the written output.

A better test of the patient's command of written language is to dictate material to be written. Letters, numbers and high and low frequency words, phrases and sentences can be dictated. A number of separate features can be analyzed (see next section) and writing to dictation probes both the patient's language and writing skills.

Another excellent writing test, to be tried only if the patient successfully writes to dictation, is to request a narrative written report on a topic such as a description of the weather, the patient's job, the route from one part of the city to another, how to change a punctured tire or prepare a meal. Narrative writing evaluates both the mechanics of writing and the ability to formulate thoughts into written language. This task is complex and often demonstrates abnormality (agraphia) in patients who have passed the tests mentioned earlier. At this level aphasics, almost without exception, will be agraphic; successful completion of a narrative report request almost excludes significant language pathology.

A number of writing tests have been used in experimental investigations of language. Most were devised for use with normal subjects and modified for experimentation on aphasics. None have proved really useful for clinical purposes. One such test, the Cloze procedure, has been used extensively (Taylor, 1953; Rutter, Draffan and Davies, 1977) and provides an example of the overall problem. In the Cloze procedure a paragraph is presented in which every fourth or fifth word is omitted; the subject's task is to provide the best possible word for the blank. The task demands overall comprehension of the mutilated paragraph plus sufficient vocabulary to select appropriate fill-ins. Most aphasics fail totally and the test can be applied only to patients suffering mild word-finding defect. As already noted, writing skills are tenuously held by most and, thus, even elementary writing tests are remarkably sensitive to brain dysfunction.

CHARACTERISTICS OF AGRAPHIA

Many analyses of writing difficulties have been offered, and a number of separable features have been suggested. Roughly, the separate features can be discussed under four major headings: 1) the quality of the handwriting (calligraphy); 2) visual spatial attributes; 3) ability to spell (orthography) and 4) appropriate choice of words (linguistic quality).

Distinguishing features in the quality of written output include the size of the individual letters, the neatness of the production and the form, whether script or block letters. Some aphasics (most often those with anterior, dominant hemisphere pathology causing a hemiplegia) produce large, messy, poorly formed block letters. Inasmuch as the written output is produced by the left hand, some of the alterations may reflect the clumsiness of the nondominant limb. As already noted, however, patients with peripheral injuries necessitating use of the nondominant limb will produce written language that is considerably less crude than the output of patients with anterior, dominant hemisphere pathology. In contrast, patients with posterior language area lesions usually produce normal-appearing, printed or script letters. In the correlation of agraphia then, the normal appearance of the calligraphy has as much localizing significance as the grossly abnormal handwriting (see Fig. 12-1). The presence of an excessive number of separations between letters or groups of letters is often noted; a tendency to segment written output has been postulated as a characteristic of nondominant hemisphere pathology, a correlation that has yet to be proved. A less common but highly noteworthy attribute is a tendency to increase the number of loops in a letter or to consecutively repeat letters made up of loops (for instance, producing extra loops in "m" or "n" or repeating the letter "e" or "o" multiple times) (see Fig. 12-1). Production of extra loops has been said to indicate frontal pathology; again, sufficient evidence is not yet

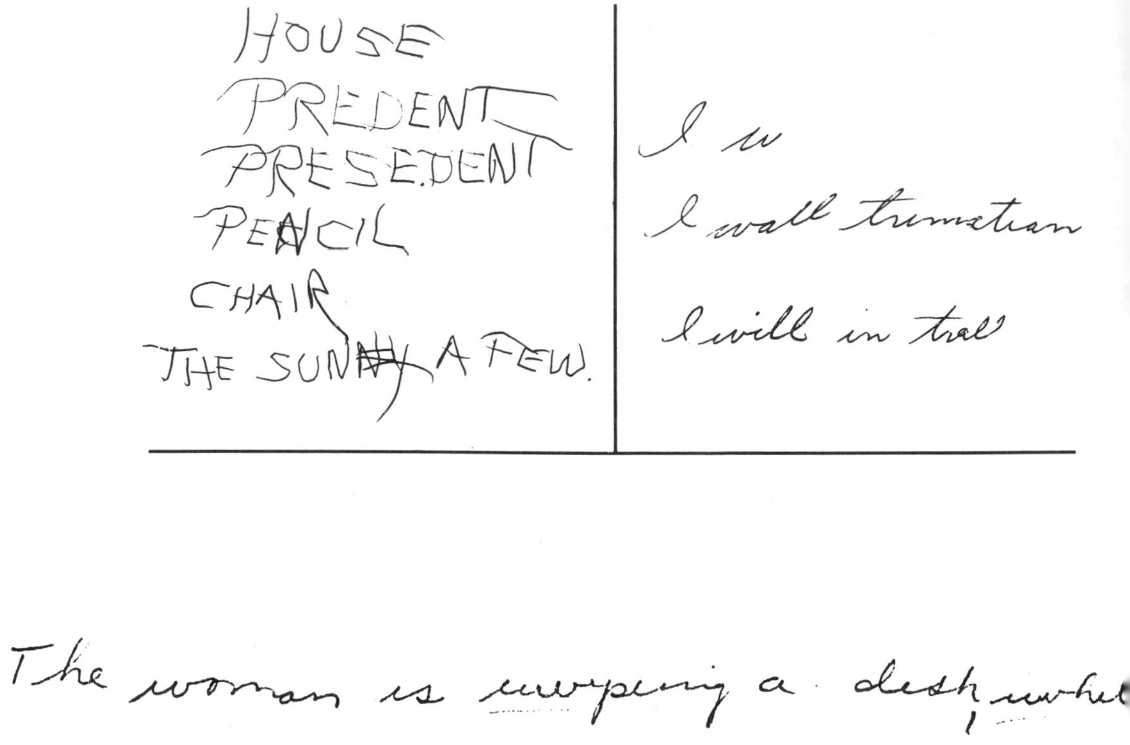

HOUSE
PREDENT
PRESEDENT
PENCIL
CHAIR
THE SUN~~DAY~~ A FEW.

I w
I wall trustian

I will in tral

The woman is sweeping a dish while
loooking out the windorow, she
forgot the water was on and
it is overrflowwang on to the floor
The little boy falls fromm a stoo
while lreyeng to git somme cookies for hi
sister and himself

Figure 12-1. A. Handwriting specimen from patient with Broca aphasia; note the big, messy letters and misspellings. B. Handwriting specimen from a patient with Wernicke aphasia showing well-formed letters but incorrect spelling and word use. C. Handwriting specimen from a patient with bifrontal damage; note multiple o's, i's, r's and m's in an otherwise adequately written description of a picture.

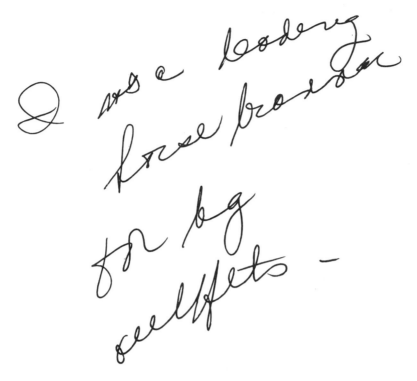

Figure 12-2. *Handwriting specimen from a patient with right parietal pathology. Note the upward slant of the lines and the enlarging left margin.*

available to accept this finding as pathognomic of frontal lobe dysfunction, but the correlation is seen in clinical practice.

Inability to maintain a normal margin for written material is commonly noted and appears to have localizing usefulness. Patients with right hemisphere pathology tend to leave a larger margin on the left, and not infrequently the margin increases as succeeding lines are written, causing the left hand margin to run diagonally across the page until the line of writing almost disappears off the right side of the page (see Fig. 12-2). In a quantitative study of graphic performance, Hecaen and Marcie (1974) found that the increasing left margin had a significant association with right hemisphere localization of pathology. Conversely, patients with left hemisphere disease may leave larger right-sided margins but this does not reach diagnostic significance.

The slant of the written line (up or down) is another noteworthy mechanical feature of handwriting. It has long been suggested that patients with right hemisphere dysfunction tend to write with an upward slant. But analysis by Hecaen's group (1974) failed to demonstrate that the direction of slant offered a reliable indicator and they concluded that it cannot be accepted as a diagnostic feature.

Spelling errors are frequent and there are suggestions that they represent pertinent indicators of the location of pathology (Kinsbourne and Rosenfield, 1974). Letter substitutions which are phonemic or clang errors (substitution of "b" or "v," etc.) can be differentiated from nonphonemic substitutions. Occasionally real but incorrect words are substituted for the target word, suggesting a correlation with the semantic type of aphasic abnormality (Simernitskaya, 1974). Letters may be reversed or misplaced; at times a word will be spelled with the correct letters but in the wrong sequence. Omission of letters occurs frequently in agraphia and letters may be repeated (perseverated) both immediately or at intervals throughout a word. While attempts have been made to correlate varieties of spelling defects with specific anatomical or psychological defects, none have proved successful.

CLINICAL CORRELATIONS OF AGRAPHIA

Among the initial excesses of cortical localization in the early days of aphasia study, was the demonstration of a cortical writing center (Exner's writing center) located in the frontal association cortex just superior to Broca's area. The correlation was logical, a motor writing center located in close proximity to the hand region of the motor cortex, just as the motor speech area lies in close proximity to the portion of the motor cortex subserving bucco-facial movements. Despite a shortage of case reports to support this correlation, Exner's center has remained in the literature for nearly a century. Many investigators have noted that agraphia occurs when this frontal area is intact, and disproving the validity of Exner's area was another strong point in the holistic argument against the localization of language function. In more recent years, however, many investigators have reported many variations in graphic breakdown and the possibility of a clinical correlation can again be suggested.

Luria (1964, 1966) suggested correlations between specific writing abnormalities and the anatomical location of cerebral disease. Three types of linguistically oriented agraphia were proposed: 1) *sensory agraphia,* usually associated with posterior-superior temporal lobe dominant hemisphere pathology and characterized by the substitution of letters which make similar sounds (clang errors); 2) *afferent agraphia,* with pathology in the dominant posterior frontal or frontal-parietal area causing substitution of incorrect letters (a literal paragraphia); 3) *sequential* or *motor agraphia* seen with dominant premotor frontal pathology in or near Broca's area, and producing abnormal sequencing of letters and sounds, frequently combining several words into a single word. In addition to the linguistic writing disturbances, Luria described two *visual-spatial* or graphic types of agraphia. One, 4) is seen with dominant parietal-occipital pathology and is characterized by written production containing misshaped letters and a tendency to mirror-write letters. A second type, 5) seen with dominant temporal occipital pathology, features substitutions by optically similar letters ("a" for "o," "m" for "n").

Hecaen has probably presented more data based on controlled studies of writing disorder than any other single investigator (Hecaen, Angelerques and

Douzinis, 1965; Dubois, Hecaen and Marcie, 1969; Hecaen and Consoli, 1973; Hecaen and Marcie, 1974). Data from these studies have been consolidated (Hecaen and Albert, 1978) and several types of agraphia (agraphic syndromes) suggested. The first is *pure agraphia,* a disorder of written language in the absence of other language disability for which a dominant frontal localization has been suggested but not conclusively proved. Under this term were included the unusual dissociations of written and oral spelling (Kinsbourne and Rosenfield, 1974), and the agraphia frequently noted in confusional states (Chedru and Geschwind, 1972). Two variations of pure agraphia, spatial-temporal disorganization and defective letter selection, were thus postulated. Another type of agraphia is *apraxic agraphia* in which written output is contaminated by distortions, inversions, reiterations and omissions of letters. Said to accompany both unilateral ideomotor apraxia and alexia, the localizations of apraxic agraphia are correlated with the localizations of these problems. A third agraphia is *spatial agraphia,* a disturbance of written output based on impaired visual-spatial perception. Additional loops are seen on appropriate letters (e.g. "m"), the written lines slant, the output is crowded to the right side of the page and individual letters are often separated. Pathology is most often found in the posterior part of the nondominant hemisphere.

Other correlations of graphic disturbances and neuroanatomical localizations have also been suggested. Parietal agraphia is similar, if not identical, to Hecaen's apraxic agraphia and is another name for agraphia of the parietal-temporal alexia syndrome. The written output in this syndrome shows a notable dichotomy; the patient is almost totally unable to produce meaningful written language to dictation or request but the copying of written language is performed adequately (often without comprehension). Another suggested form of agraphia has been called callosal agraphia (or hemiagraphia). The patient with a total (or even an anterior two-thirds) callosal section may write adequately with the dominant hand while failing totally to produce meaningful written language with the other hand (Geschwind and Kaplan, 1962; Sperry and Gazzaniga, 1967). It is claimed that patients with a callosal separation will copy better with the nondominant hand while other writing skills are performed only by the dominant hand (Bogen, 1969). This dyscopia-dysgraphia dichotomy has not been consistently demonstrated.

As the foregoing pages attest, the clinical abnormalities of writing are complex and have resisted rigid anatomical-psychological correlations. Nonetheless, data are available that demonstrate a number of distinctive variations within agraphia and at least crude anatomical correlations can be suggested. For purposes of simplicity (and honesty) only three variations will be outlined here although it is admitted that a number of additional separations appear genuine. To maintain the pattern used in the discussion of alexia, neuroanatomical terminology will be used.

Dominant Frontal (Anterior) Agraphia

Most often seen in patients with hemiplegia involving the dominant hemisphere, the written output by the nonpreferred hand is large and messy and spelling is poor, showing either omissions or phonetic spelling. The written output is limited to individual, substantive words, and, if a full sentence is requested, omission of the short, grammatical words is noted, an agrammatism in writing.

Dominant Parietal-Temporal (Posterior) Agraphia

In this disorder the mechanics of writing are normal or nearly so but there are notable errors in spelling (omission, reversals or substitution of letters) and the words are often segmented. Some patients substitute full words (verbal paragraphia) and many produce wordy but empty writing, similar to the empty output of a patient with severe anomia. These patients characteristically have no hemiplegia but may have other lateralizing neurologic defects. Most often, the dominant (right) hand is used to produce this agraphic output.

Nondominant Agraphia

Most commonly associated with posterior right hemisphere defects causing visual-spatial disturbance, this variation of agraphia is entirely mechanical and does not have the aphasic qualities of the other two. The script or block letters are formed adequately but there is a tendency for the written line to slant upwards and for the left margin to be larger and increase in size with subsequent lines. The graphic disturbance may be sufficiently severe to produce a true impairment of the ability to communicate by writing and thus qualify as a variety of agraphia.

While the above classification of types of agraphia is admittedly incomplete and does not encompass all discernable variations of graphic disturbance, it is sufficiently simple and specific to be useful for the practicing clinician. Hopefully, future investigations on writing disturbance will provide additional practical information to this initial outline.

13

Related Syndromes and a Postscript

A number of conditions crop up in clinical practice which closely resemble one or more of the traditioanl aphasia syndromes but involve only a single, language-related modality, not language function as a whole. Whether these conditions truly deserve inclusion with the aphasias is open to question, but they so closely resemble and are so frequently confused with aphasic disorders that they deserve discussion in the same context. Several entities of this nature have already been discussed. Occipital alexia (alexia without agraphia) (see Ch. 11) is a classic example of a disturbance in which only a single modality, the ability to visualize language information, is abnormal. In occipital alexia the written communication signs are received but there is failure to transmit them to an area capable of interpretation, producing a distinct syndrome. It seems doubtful that this syndrome should be classed as aphasic, inasmuch as language function remains intact for all activities except the transmission of visual language symbols. In a similar vein, some of the varieties of word-finding defect (anomia) are best classed as nonaphasic conditions (Benson, 1979). "Pure" anomia appears to involve only a single aspect of a single function, naming on confrontation, and doesn't necessarily indicate aphasia. In addition, some degree of word-finding problem is present (and may be prominent) in many types of dementia, even in the early stages when the patient has no other indication of a language disturbance. Several other "anomias" appear in "nonaphasia" circumstances; for instance, the "nonaphasic" anomia of the acute confusional state or the pseudoanomia of an hysterical reaction are not, strictly speaking, language disorders.

The disorders to be described in this chapter share this trait of an isolated modality function disturbance and are routinely difficult to separate from aphasic conditions. While each is comparatively rare in pure state, in practice these problems are often mixed with other language or nonlanguage disturbances, producing seriously confusing combinations.

APHEMIA

This syndrome has been given a number of different names but none has achieved general acceptance. Aphemia was the term originally used by Broca to describe all language disturbances but he later accepted the term *aphasia* promoted by Trousseau (1864); Bastian (1887) used aphemia to denote a specific syndrome and subsequent authors have used *pure word dumbness, pure motor aphasia, cortical anarthria* and *subcortical motor aphasia* to identify the same collection of findings. We will use Bastian's term but recognize that aphemia has not acheieved widespread acceptance. On the other hand, the syndrome is unique and does enjoy fairly widespread recognition.

The clinical picture of aphemia is distinct. Initially the patient becomes mute, usually acutely, and temporarily is totally unable to express himself or herself vocally. In contrast, the aphemic patient can use written language quite well to express his or her ideas. Eventually there is recovery from the mute state, sometimes within a few days but more often weeks go by before verbalization begins to return. During this period the patient becomes adept at writing his or her verbal output. When vocalization does return for the aphemic the output is hypophonic, slow, breathy and so poorly articulated as to be almost incomprehensible. Careful observation, however, reveals that the syntactical structure is intact, even in the earliest stages of vocal recovery. Language evaluation shows that the ability to comprehend spoken language is fully intact. While both repetition and naming are failed because they demand vocalization, the patient can read and write without difficulty. The written output tends to be complete with normal grammatic structure and a full lexicon. Aphemic patients often carry a pad of paper, and although unable to vocalize usefully they can communicate fully in writing. Primary laryngeal pathology must be ruled out.

A right-sided hemiplegia or paralysis is often present at the onset of aphemia but characteristically disappears quickly, leaving the patient without discernable neurologic findings (paresis, sensory loss or visual field disturbance). One neurologic finding, bucco-facial apraxia, can be demonstrated in many cases. While not constantly present, many patients with aphemia have distinct difficulty performing on command such acts as whistling, coughing, blowing, sucking and winking. In contrast, they have no difficulty performing limb activities such as making a fist, waving goodbye, beckoning or imitating the use of a toothbrush or comb.

In aphemia the communication disturbance appears to involve only verbal output and can be considered a speech problem rather than an impairment of language. For diagnostic purposes, however, the clinician must consider aphemia when evaluating anterior aphasia. Not only can aphemia be mistaken for Broca aphasia if sufficient examination is not performed, but it seems apparent that an overlap can exist between aphemia and all varieties of anterior aphasia. In fact some suggest that the aphemic condition merely represents the least severe (or best recovered) variation of anterior aphasia (Mohr et al, 1978). The consistent description of aphemia in the early stages and the distinct clinical picture (particularly the hypophonic but syntactically intact output) speak against this suggestion but an aphemia-like condition does appear in some cases of recovered Broca aphasia. Aphemia improves to useful language output, but a residual dysprosody almost invariably remains. Not infrequently the altered speech pattern suggests a foreign accent (Monrod-Krohn, 1947).

Most cases of aphemia follow cerebral vascular problems. Mohr et al (1975) suggest that emboli commonly cause aphemia and consideration of this diagnosis warrants a diligent search for a source of embolization. Other recorded cases, however, have followed large infarctions, hematomas and trauma. Most confirmed cases have been localized by autopsy (see Weisenburg and McBride, 1935 for a review of early cases) but they can also be localized by CAT scan and radioisotope brain scan (Brown, 1972).

Only a few cases of aphemia have come to autopsy but they have revealed interesting findings. Based on limited autopsy material, Bastian (1898) suggested that aphemia occurred when pathology undercut the cortex of Broca's area, leaving the frontal cortex intact but isolating it from its normal outflow channels via the internal capsule or across the corpus callosum to the opposite hemisphere. Bastian's book details several cases of aphemia with autopsy study, at least one of which fulfills the neuroanatomical criteria of a subcortical motor aphasia. Other authors, however, have suggested that aphemia may result from direct involvement of Broca's area itself (Souques, 1928), and recent reports by Mohr and his colleagues (1975, 1978) describe several cases with verbal output resembling aphemia in which the pathology directly involved the cortex of Broca's area. At present it is best to state that aphemia may occur with either direct involvement of Broca's area or damage to the subcortical tissues immediately below this area.

In addition to aphemia and primary laryngeal pathology, mutism can result from disorder in a number of other cerebral locations. Acute involvement of the dominant hemisphere supplementary motor area characteristically produces mutism followed by hypophonic but semantically and grammatically intact verbal output. Neurosurgeons have recorded this syndrome frequently, particularly following removal of a frontal parasaggital meningioma. Additional sources of mutism and a fuller description of the disorder are presented in Chapter 15.

Aphemia is not common but is a clinically separate entity that can be diagnosed with certainty in many instances. The importance of correct diagnosis lies in the somewhat better prognosis, the need for a radically different therapeutic approach (primarily therapy for speech) and, at least in some cases, the need to alert the clinician to the possibility of embolic disease.

APRAXIA OF SPEECH

Closely related to and frequently combined with aphemia is a condition characterized by disturbed articulatory motor control and often called apraxia. Unfortunately, apraxia is a badly misused term in neurology and the various meanings of apraxia applied to verbal expression not only reflect this missue but serve to compound an already difficult problem. A full review of the use of the term apraxia is beyond the scope of this volume. (Ch. 16 presents a limited discussion) but apraxia is used so frequently in discussions of aphasic (or nonaphasic) verbal output that it deserves comment here.

In his classic papers on apraxia, Liepmann (1900, 1905) suggested that a similar disturbance, a variety of motor apraxia, could affect speech. Liepmann did not describe any clinical findings of language apraxia but over the years the term has been used extensively, particularly by speech pathologists. Unfortunately, several different definitions or meanings of the term have evolved causing both controversy and confusion. The term has been sufficiently misused to warrant a major address at an annual meeting of the American Speech and Hearing Association entitled "Apraxia of Speech; 107 Years of Terminological Confusion" (Darley, 1968).

A review of the definitions of apraxia in reference to language and aphasia as they appear in the current literature reveals four distinctly different clinical dysfunctions.

Verbal apraxia is the most widely used term to denote apraxia as a form of speech pathology. It is routinely used by many speech pathologists (Sarno and Sands, 1970; Trost and Canter, 1974) to represent the articulatory abnormalities present in cases of motor or expressive aphasia. Operationally, verbal apraxia has been described as a sparse verbal output, poorly articulated, produced with effort and with abnormal phrase length and melody. This is a broad description and contains most of the features used to describe nonfluent aphasic output.

The term *bucco-lingual* (oral apraxia) (Nathan, 1947) has been used more often by Europeans, usually implicating the articulatory abnormalities described as verbal apraxia but emphasizing the loss of fine control of the lips, tongue, palate, etc. that can occur with brain damage. The term *cortical dysarthria* used by Whitty (1964) and Bay (1964) refers to an apraxia of speech mechanisms although Bay clearly describes this as a motor disturbance of the articulatory musculature plus impairment of tongue movements.

Apraxia of speech has been used in several ways. In one form, apraxia of speech is used to characterize patients who are unable to speak (clearly) but have no other language problem (Johns and Darley, 1970). Not only can these patients comprehend spoken language normally, but they can also express themselves in written language. In its pure state this is a notably rare disturbance that has been called aphemia in this chapter.

A second description of apraxia of speech emphasizes the lack of a consistent defect in articulation (Darley, 1975). All phonemes can be correctly produced at times but under circumstances of specific language demand the substitution of incorrect phonemes (literal paraphasia) occurs frequently but inconsistently. This disorder is most clearly illustrated by a failure to repeat spoken language with many more errors occurring with repetition than with conversational language use. This description is similar if not identical to the output characteristics of conduction aphasia (see Ch. 7). It should be noted that the second definition of apraxia of speech is consistent with both Leipmann's use of apraxia and most current usages of the term (Geschwind, 1965).

Apraxia of speech is rare as a pure entity, occurring most often with aphasia, generally a Broca aphasia. Specific speech characteristics have been outlined to differentiate apraxia of speech (cortical dysarthria) from the dysarthria of subcortical brain disturbance (Trost and Canter, 1974). These include: 1) inconsistency of articulatory errors; 2) substitutions rather than distortions of individual phonemes; 3) lack of major neuromotor impairment in the vocal musculature; 4) greater difficulty producing initial than following phonemes; 5) a significant latency in speech production; 6) actual alterations rather than mere simplifications of the phonemes when making errors and 7) patient awareness of error production.

While apraxia of speech is a term used commonly by speech pathologists, the meaning has proved difficult for neurologists to understand. In general, apraxia of speech appears to represent a disturbance of the motor programming of speech as noted in some types of aphasia. It must be emphasized that apraxia of speech, as defined, is independent and separate from aphasia, a disturbance of language (Critchley, 1952; Bay, 1964; Darley, 1975). In this respect, apraxia of speech is a true speech disturbance in the sense outlined in Chapter 1 in contrast to aphasia, a disturbance of language.

PURE WORD DEAFNESS

Another striking example of single modality involvement has been called pure word deafness as well as verbal auditory agnosia (see Ch. 16 for a discussion of nonverbal auditory agnosia). In this condition the patient cannot comprehend spoken language, is "word deaf" but can read without difficulty, both out loud and for comprehension. While many descriptions of pure word deafness have appeared in the literature (Liepmann and Storck, 1902; Schuster and Taterka, 1926; Klein and Harper, 1956; Gazzaniga et al, 1973), the syndrome is by no means common.

Although patients with pure word deafness are said to have fully normal spontaneous speech, most display some degree of language output disorder at the onset. Both literal and verbal paraphasia have been reported but the output problems decrease with time and eventually disappear Patients with long-standing pure word deafness show little or no discernable problem with verbal output. From the onset these patients do not understand spoken language and are unable to repeat; if recovery occurs, the ability to repeat improves along with comprehension. Several reports document that the speed of language presentation affects comprehension in pure word deafness (Goldstein, quoting Schmitt, 1948; Albert and Bear, 1974). Thus if words are presented slowly, the patient with pure word deafness may comprehend fairly well; if presented at a normal or rapid sqeed, however, the patient will not comprehend. Other reports describe patients who perceive vowels and/or consonants but not entire words (Ziehl, 1896; Henneberg, 1918; Bonvicini, 1929) or some words but not vowels or consonants (Goldstein, 1948). Patients with pure word deafness have little difficulty with naming, reading or writing; all language functions except auditory comprehension are performed with ease.

Pure word deafness is differentiated from Wernicke aphasia by the preservation of reading ability in the former, and to a lesser degree by the comparatively normal spontaneous output, good naming and normal writing of pure word deafness. Many individual cases fall between "pure" word deafness and "pure" Wernicke aphasia, exhibiting some characteristics of both. Many posterior aphasics have greater difficulty comprehending oral than written language but show significant difficulty in both. Others have the opposite problem, greater word blindness than word deafness. To be called "pure" word deafness, the reading ability must be essentially intact and auditory comprehension severely defective, which is a striking combination.

As a rule there are no associated neurologic findings accompanying pure word deafness. Unilateral paresis and hemisensory abnormality do not occur (or disappear rapidly) and only rarely is a superior quadrantanopsia reported. Of most significance is the presence of normal hearing. Some reports describe an initial "cortical" deafness followed by either nonverbal auditory agnosia (Albert et al, 1972) or verbal auditory agnosia (Goldstein, 1974). For a diagnosis of pure word deafness, careful audiometric testing must demonstrate no significant defect. The patient can hear the language sounds but they remain meaningless, as if spoken in a foreign tongue. Most localization has been by autopsy but both CAT scan and radioisotope scans have been used effectively to indicate the locale of pathology causing pure word deafness.

Studies of pure word deafness have demonstrated both unilateral and bilateral temporal lesions (Barrett, 1910; Schuster and Taterka, 1926). The unilateral lesions are consistently located deep in the dominant posterior temporal lobe, apparently affecting either Heschl's gyrus or the fibres streaming into this primary auditory cortex (Gazzaniga et al, 1973). Wernicke's area, the dominant auditory association center, is not involved. In those cases with bilateral lesions the pathology characteristically involves the mid portion of the first temporal gyrus of both hemispheres. Again Wernicke's area, specifically the posterior portion of the first temporal gyrus of the dominant hemisphere, is spared. The etiology has been variable. Tumor, trauma (Goldstein, 1948) and infection (Goldstein, Brown and Hollander, 1975) have been reported but vascular accidents are certainly the most frequent cause of the unilateral and almost the exclusive source of the bilateral temporal pathology producing pure word deafness.

Pure word deafness is not a true disturbance of language capability either. These patients handle written language in a normal manner and produce grammatically and semantically full verbal output. It appears that the ability to deliver the auditory language stimuli to the cortical area mandatory for language interpretation is defective, a sensory transmission problem rather than a language disturbance. Symptomatically, pure word deafness resembles deafness more than aphasia. While it should not be classed as a form of aphasia, pure word deafness must be considered when aphasia is suspected, and even more than aphemia or occipital alexia, pure word deafness is present as a significant contaminant of many posterior aphasic disorders.

NONAPHASIC MISNAMING

A qualitatively distinct naming disturbance has been described in many articles by Weinstein and his colleagues (Weinstein and Kahn, 1952; Weinstein and Keller, 1973) and deserves consideration as a word-finding defect. Originally, the misnaming was considered a form of paraphasia, and by implication the disturbance was classed as a form of aphasia. Comparative studies of the phenomenon, however, indicated that many of the word substitutions were motivated and apparently unrelated to the semantic paraphasias of posterior aphasia and are better described as nonaphasic misnaming.

Most of the patients with nonaphasic misnaming described by the authors were acutely ill, often in a state of reduced consciousness due to widespread cerebral dysfunction (e.g. increased intracranial pressure, metabolic encephalopathy, posttraumatic twilight state, intoxication). While the nonaphasic misnaming phenomenon in an obtunded patient is usually easy to distinguish from aphasic anomia in a clear mental state, the two conditions frequently overlap. Not only can nonaphasic misnaming occur in an apparently alert patient or aphasia in an obtunded patient but a brain-injured individual may present aphasic and nonaphasic naming problems simultaneously. Weinstein emphasized that the misnamed words are characteristically related to stress or illness; items or activities referring to hospitalization, such as the name of the hospital, a thermometer, or urinal, were likely to be misnamed whereas neutral items were named correctly. In some instances a misnaming error appears confabulatory and leads to a series of confabulations, related to an original misnaming. Thus the patient who calls the doctor a bus driver may misidentify items of hospital furniture as portions of a bus.

Along with the misnaming, other unique symptoms are frequent in these patients, such as disorientation, denial of illness and reduplication of place or person (for instance the patient may insist that there are two hospitals with the same name, one in its proper location, the other located nearer the patient's locale) (Weinstein and Cole, 1963). Nonaphasic misnaming characteristically occurs in patients whose decreased level of conscious awareness interferes with attention and/or memory; however, both the amount and the character of the misnaming are very different in this disorder from any naming problems seen in amnesia such as Korsakoff's psychosis (see Ch. 16).

Clinical studies reveal that most patients with nonaphasic misnaming have "diffuse" cerebral dysfunction, even in the presence of focal brain abnormality (Weinstein and Kahn, 1955). This was clearly demonstrated by the EEG which routinely showed bilateral slowing, often superimposed over a focal EEG abnormality. Right hemisphere focus is more common than left in reported cases, but misnaming can occur with a focus in either hemisphere and occurs, not infrequently in the absence of a demonstrable EEG focus (Weinstein and Kahn, 1955).

Nonaphasic misnaming is usually a symptom of an acute confusional syndrome, and as such it is almost always transient. The confabulatory character of the misnaming, the presence of "diffuse" bilateral dysfunction rather than left focal abnormality and, possibly, the psychodynamic nature of the naming errors, all imply that nonaphasic misnaming differs from true aphasia. The condition, however, is easily mistaken for aphasia and, not infrequently, the two disorders coexist. Nonaphasic misnaming is worthy of strong consideration when abnormal verbal output is present in a patient with a depressed state of consciousness.

POSTSCRIPT ON THE SYNDROMES OF APHASIA

Better than a dozen separable aphasia syndromes have been outlined, and in addition a number of closely related but not truly aphasic disorders have been described. Each entity can, with greater or lesser ease, be distinguished from the others, both clinically and neuroanatomically. However, even utilizing this large number of syndromes, only about half of the cases of aphasia seen routinely in a clinical practice can clearly be placed into one or another of the syndromes and even this figure is dependent upon some degree of diagnostic flexibility. Rigidly exacting examiners will find even fewer individual cases that completely fulfill prerequisites for any one of these syndrome labels.

Table 13-1 graphically demonstrates this diagnostic problem by tabulating individual patients admitted to the Aphasia Research Center of the Boston Veterans Administration Hospital and subsequently presented at the Thursday Morning Aphasia Conference over a period of almost a decade (1964–73). Each patient was evaluated by a team of examiners (neurologists, psychologists, speech therapists, linguists) with each specialist seeking information germane to their particular interest. Following presentation the diagnosis was discussed, and whenever possible the locus of involvement predicted by aphasia type was correlated with nonlanguage localizing information. Anatomical correlation was high (almost 90 percent) (Benson and Patten, 1967) but an exact syndrome diagnosis was only possible in 59 percent. Over 40 percent of these carefully studied cases could not be placed in a specific syndrome.

What is the cause of this low yield of syndrome diagnoses? Any number of reasons are apparent and the problem deserves discussion. One obvious complication stems from the presence of multiple and/or extensive lesions involving several anatomically significant areas and causing mixed clinical pictures. The aphasia syndromes described in the previous chapters have been observed in individuals suffering comparatively focal hemispheric pathology. It would be anticipated that multiple lesions, or pathology extending over a broad cortical area, would obscure the clinical features of the syndromes. Both conditions, multiple pathological sites and large lesions, are common in neurological practice and make syndrome diagnosis difficult.

Similarly, an aphasia-producing lesion is frequently superimposed on a brain made abnormal by previous damage (arteriosclerotic, degenerative, surgical, traumatic, etc.) creating complex aphasia pictures. For instance, one common clinical picture is superimposition of an aphasia-producing lesion on a

Table 13-1. THURSDAY CONFERENCE DIAG-
NOSES, APHASIA RESEARCH CENTER, BOSTON

Syndrome	I	II	Total
Broca	69	37	106
Wernicke	53	28	81
Conduction	23	19	42
Transcortical motor	10	4	14
Transcortical sensory	2	4	6
Mixed transcortical	2	3	5
Global	28	56	84
Anomic	53	26	79
Alexia with agraphia	9	2	11
Alexia without agraphia	5	0	5
Pure word deafness	4	0	4
Aphemia	5	2	7
TOTAL	263	181	444

I and II refer to the certainty of the syndrome diagnosis; I indicates most certain diagnosis and II less definite diagnosis. Note
that these results do not reflect the frequency of varieties of
aphasia in clinical practice. These cases were chosen from the
inpatient population of a rehabilitation service and include an
excessive number of chronic and severe problems. Other aphasia
populations should have different frequencies of the various syndromes.

dementing disorder or some other extraneous process producing a syndrome
that defies localization. Chapter 16 outlines a number of brain damage disturbances frequently associated with aphasia to produce complicated clinical pictures. The presence of such problems as amnesia, confusional state, agnosia,
right hemisphere damage and major subcortical symptomatology severely
complicate the clinical picture of aphasia. Nonetheless, even in these complex
situations, specific aphasia syndromes can often be discerned, albeit somewhat
obscured.

Finally, it seems probable that future studies will demonstrate additional,
more clearly delineated aphasia syndromes associated with specific localizations and that some of the current diagnostic indecision will be corrected. To
some degree, such a step is occurring at present with the consideration of the
subcortical types of language disorder. In view of the many potential complicating factors, however, it is not at all surprising that pure examples of the aphasic
syndromes are not common, and in fact it is remarkable that the recognizable
syndromes shine through as often as they do. The language disabilities of
aphasia appear to be strong clinical signs.

Is the study of the aphasia syndromes of any real value? There appears to be
a comparatively firm neuroanatomical basis for many of the language defect

syndromes but whether this correlation is of value for either clinical or research purposes may be questioned. For the practicing neurologist, at the time of this writing, the localization of aphasia-producing lesions is admittedly of limited and mostly academic value. Neurodiagnostic tools such as the CAT scan, arteriography, radioisotope scan, EEG and others have become the standard for cerebral localization. Most research scientists laboring in the field of language have worked without concern about anatomical correlations for years; only recently has an increasing realization of the focal nature of language functions developed, leading a number of language investigators to rediscover the aphasia syndromes. Similarly, the language therapist has traditionally worked with little consideration for the formal aphasic syndromes, preferring to treat each aphasic patient as an individual problem. Recent advances in language therapy techniques suggest that some varieties (syndromes) of aphasia respond best to certain techniques, and future advances may well demonstrate even greater specificity between the variety of aphasia and the most favorable treatment technique. If such a step occurs, aphasia therapy will be closer to working on a medical model, making a diagnosis from the available clinical data and selecting the optimum form of therapy for that diagnosis. Obviously, the language information outlined in the aphasia syndromes would be of considerable consequence in this approach.

The remaining chapters will discuss aphasia and related conditions from other viewpoints but will constantly refer back to and utilize the foundation of the syndrome approach. Syndromes are, by the definition offered earlier, artificial, but they appear to be of continuing and increasing importance in the understanding of aphasia. Quite possibly the day will come when the understanding of language-processing will be sufficiently sophisticated to allow abandonment of the syndrome approach. Until such a time, however, it is foolish to ignore any source of information. The clinical descriptions of the aphasia syndromes have remained remarkably consistent for over a century, a period that has seen the passing of dozens of brilliant theories of language function, and the syndrome approach still offers a reliable avenue to language study.

14

Lateralization of Language

Many of the syndromes discussed in the previous chapters date from the 19th century and were the products of a golden age of clinical-pathological correlations prevalent in continental Europe. Correlation of the language syndromes and the gross anatomical findings of neuropathological studies showed acceptable consistency (and still do), but attempts to correlate less clinical topics (i.e. ideation, verbal imagery, reading) were much less successful. In fact, a number of the hypothesized language centers (such as Exner's writing center) cannot be substantiated. Many of the early correlations of individual language functions with neuroanatomy were far too specific, were based on insufficient evidence, were both misleading and incorrect and have been justifiably criticized. The neuroanatomical localization of individual language functions became, and remains, suspect.

This unfortunate state derived, at least in part, from overzealousness on the part of the early scientists and in part from the limited resources available to them for reference, but in the main this stemmed from simplified, concrete interpretations of language functions. Attempts to localize ideas, images, verbal memories, etc. were doomed to failure just as isolated centers for speech, for reading, writing, calculating and others could never be fully substantiated. Those 19th century physicians who adequately recognized the breadth of the problems under discussion avoided didactic localizations (Hughlings Jackson, Arnold Pick and many others). Much of the criticism of the diagram-making localizationists was valid and led to the holistic attitude toward the brain's function most fully developed by Lashley (1929) and others (Chapman and Wolff, 1959). In no aspect of aphasia study was the shift away from strict clinical localization toward a more general, holistic viewpoint more deserved than in the studies of individual language functions.

There are many valid reasons to be wary of anatomical-clinical correlations of specific language functions. First, there is considerable variation in the development of intellectual functions among individual humans. No absolute proof exists showing that one neuroanatomic area subserves the same function in different individuals. Significant variations in cortical neuroanatomy are regularly noted and a given anatomical structure may appear to underlie quite different functions in different individuals, based on either developmental or experimental background.

A second important point is that most of the language activities that have been discussed are too crudely defined for scientific correlation. The terminology promoted by most students of language (philosophers, psychologists, linguists, etc.) is in a state of constant alteration; descriptive language terms attain only limited specificity, most existing in the rarified and inconsistent air of intellectual discussion, and by the time they become widely recognized their meanings are muddied.

In this same vein, neuroanatomical localization remains crude. Study of living aphasic patients, a necessity for intensive language testing, limits localization to indirect techniques such as isotope brain scans, electroencephalograms and CAT scans. These tools provide crude information but are incapable of exact localization. Even autopsy examination often leaves questions about the specificity of localization. This very real problem of lesion localization in patients with aphasia is discussed further in Chapter 5.

The most pertinent of all difficulties plaguing the correlation of specific language functions with neuroanatomy, however, lies in the generally poor quality of clinical and anatomical examinations given to most aphasics. The strongest criticism of the clinical-anatomical correlations has always come from individuals who are incompetent at both clinical and anatomical studies. Actually, few individuals are sufficiently sophisticated to discuss advanced levels of both neuroanatomy and language evaluation. Those who do have these skills are the ones who report considerable success in demonstrating clinical-anatomical correlations. The success of clinical-anatomical correlation is far greater when well-trained individuals perform the study. Expertise in cortical neuroanatomy is not essential to the study of language, but criticism of the neuroanatomical correlates of aphasia should be reserved for those who have both knowledge and experience in the subject.

Against this background, what is known and/or suggested about the anatomical localization of individual language functions will be reviewed. At best, the correlations must remain vague. The major language categories under consideration are probably incorrect (or at least overinclusive) and our anatomical knowledge remains crude. Even so, some correlations of language function and neuroanatomical localization have been established and a number of other correlations can be proposed based on existing data. Such anatomical-clinical correlations would appear to offer an opportunity for advancement in the study of language function.

In the next chapter localization of a number of crude language functions and their neuroanatomical correlations will be reviewed. In the present chapter, discussion will be limited to the most dramatic and totally accepted of all neuroanatomical-functional correlations, that of the lateralization of language function to a single cerebral hemisphere.

CEREBRAL DOMINANCE FOR LANGUAGE

Almost the first and certainly the most striking of the neuroanatomical correlates of aphasia was the observation by Broca in 1865 that almost all patients who lost speech following brain damage had pathology involving the left hemisphere. Similar pathology, symmetrically placed in the right hemisphere, was rarely associated with language disturbance. This observation had evidently been made earlier (Dax, 1836; Benton, 1964) but remained unknown until the pronouncement by Broca. With few exceptions, subsequent observations have confirmed this totally unexpected observation. Lateralization of language function to a single cerebral hemisphere is so generally accepted now that we often fail to realize the unnatural state that it represents, an asymmetry in function by an apparently symmetrical organ. The anomaly of this functional asymmetry becomes apparent when we remember that while animal bodies contain many paired organs (kidneys, lungs, eyes, etc.), only in the human brain does one organ subserve a major function while the matched organ on the other side does not serve the function at all. If, as now seems possible, a number of additional higher mental functions also have unilateral localization in the cerebral hemispheres, this observation by Broca may well rank with the other great discoveries of the 19th century (such as the concepts of evolution and the unconscious).

It is often stated that better than 99 percent of all right-handed individuals have language function exclusively in the left hemisphere; in other words they become aphasic following an appropriately placed left hemisphere lesion but suffer no aphasia after damage to the identical anatomical area of the right hemisphere. This hemispheric lateralization of behavioral function has been called *dominance*. It now appears that similar hemispheric dominances may exist for functions other than language but the unilateral localization of language function to the left hemisphere in right-handed individuals is certainly the most dramatic, absolute and fully accepted example of cerebral dominance.

While the lateralization of language function in a right-handed individual is strongly to the left hemisphere, left-handed individuals (better identified as nonright handers to denote the incompleteness of their lateralized functions) do not fit this pattern clearly. Many studies based on aphasia in nonright handers suggest that left hemisphere language dominance is still more common than right (approximately a 60–40 split) (Goodglass and Quadfasel, 1954; Roberts, 1969), but the picture is not actually that clear. It appears that most nonright-handed individuals have considerable language function in both hemispheres (bilateral language dominance) (Luria, 1970; Gloning, 1977). The bilaterality of language function in nonright handers is readily apparent from two observations, the greater frequency of aphasia following brain injury in nonright handers (Gloning et al, 1969) and their better recovery rate (Luria, 1970). A third suggestion, that stuttering is a product of mixed language laterality, is far less widely accepted but receives some support (see Ch. 16). Whether some degree of bilaterality of language function is more common in the right-handed population than usually suggested is debated, but the striking finding of severe aphasia following left hemisphere damage compared to the lack of significant language disturbance after right hemisphere damage in this group is totally accepted.

Tests of Hemispheric Dominance

The determination of which hemisphere is language-dominant in an individual patient has proved to be difficult. If the patient is right-handed the probability that the left hemisphere is dominant is excellent (better than 99 to 1 odds are difficult to beat). If left-handed, or even if there is a family history of left-handedness, the possibility of mixed laterality demands consideration. Obviously, the presence of unilateral hemispheric damage, with or without aphasia, provides useful information but may be misleading. In particular, a dominant left hemisphere may have significant pathology without aphasia occurring. A test for determining the language-dominant hemisphere that does not demand structural brain damage is needed. Two techniques are presently used for this determination but neither has proved fully satisfactory.

The carotid amytal test, introduced by Wada and Rasmussen (1960), is performed by injecting fast-acting barbiturate into one of the internal carotid arteries, effectively but transiently paralyzing the ipsilateral cerebral hemisphere with only minimal effect on the other hemisphere. If the drugged hemisphere is language-dominant, the patient will develop aphasia in addition to a contralateral hemiplegia; if the hemisphere is not dominant there will be hemiplegia but no aphasia. This technique has been widely used and reported by many investigators (Milner, 1974; Milner, Branch and Rasmussen, 1964; Serafatinides, 1966; Kløve, Grabow and Trites, 1969), but it has significant limitations. Foremost is the danger to the patient resulting from injecting needles and foreign material (contrast medium) into the cerebral vascular system. The currently preferred technique of arterial catherization, utilizing the femoral artery or some other distant vessel, increases the safety of the carotid amytal test somewhat but still represents some risk to the patient and, therefore, limits its usefulness as a diagnostic procedure. Most investigators reserve carotid amytal injection for patients scheduled to undergo carotid angiography for diagnostic reasons, a rapidly decreasing group since the advent of computerized tomography.

Another, much safer evaluation of hemispheric language dominance, called dichotic listening (Broadbent, 1971; Kimura, 1967) has been introduced in recent years. Patients are given ear phones that carry separate messages to the right and left ears and, theoretically, to the contralateral hemispheres. If different messages (usually short lists of digits) are presented to the two ears simultaneously there is a tendency for extinction of one set of stimuli. It is surmised that the dominant hemisphere perceives best and the message from the right ear will be the one most often repeated after dichotic stimulation. Unfortunately, with concentration, most normal adults can and often do overcome the tendency to extinguish the signal from the nondominant ear and confusing results appear. Dichotic listening, when given to large groups, particularly of young children, provides statistically significant evidence of language dominance in the left hemisphere (Kimura, 1967). For individuals, however, the test has not proved sufficiently reliable to be acceptable as the indicator of the dominant hemisphere. The unreliability of dichotic listening testing is increased if pathology affects either hemisphere. Pathology involving the right hemisphere may produce a considerable extinction of left ear stimulation but even this is not consistent (probably based on the location of pathology within the hemisphere). Even more confusing is the demonstration that pathology in the left hemisphere can and does produce extinction of signals coming to the left ear, to the right ear or to neither (Sparks, Goodglass and Nickel, 1970). Again, this variability appears to depend upon the anatomical locus of the pathology. Interruption of pathways from the right hemisphere auditory area to the language area of the left hemisphere can produce left-ear extinction whereas interruption of the signals coming directly from the right ear can produce a right-ear extinction (see Fig. 14-1).

An accurate, safe test of language dominance is still needed. There can be

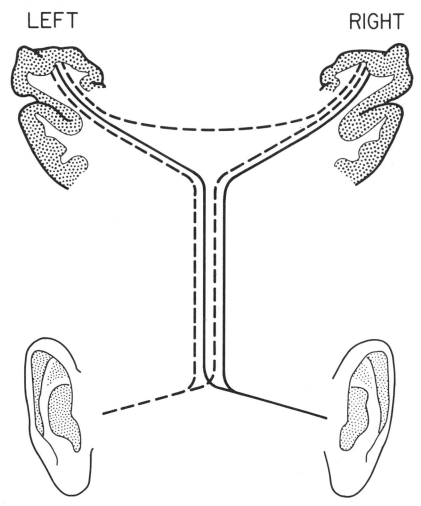

LEFT   RIGHT

Figure 14-1. *Schematic representation of the major auditory pathways. Left hemisphere pathology involving the transcallosal pathway will produce a left ear extinction to double simultaneous stimulation. Involvement of the lower pathways on the left side will produce right ear extinction. See text for additional description of dichotic listening.*

no doubt, however, that hemispheric dominance for language exists and offers an obvious and important neuroanatomical-clinical correlation.

Neuroanatomical Basis of Cerebral Dominance

What, if any, anatomical structural differences underlie this dramatic functional asymmetry? The two hemispheres have always appeared to be identical anatomical objects, essentially mirror-images of each other, and a functional asymmetry without concomitant anatomical difference has been difficult to explain. In recent years, a number of separate studies have demonstrated subtle but nonetheless real anatomical asymmetries between the two hemispheres. Yakovlev and Rakic (1966) demonstrated asymmetrical crossing of pyramidal motor fibres in the medulla oblongata (decussation of the pyramids). Motor fibres coming from the left hemisphere begin to decussate higher and cross more completely than those from the right. Thus the right cortico-spinal tract has a greater neuronal supply, quite possibly a significant factor in the superiority of the right hand for performing fine digital activities. McCrae, Branch and Milner (1968) demonstrated an asymmetry in the size of the occipital horns of the lateral ventricles, the left being both longer and broader. This finding has been confirmed by many investigators using the CAT scan and would suggest more subcortical white matter occupying the posterior part of the right hemisphere, consistent with the dominance for visual functions of the posterior portion of the right hemisphere. Using the angiogram LeMay and Culebras (1972) demonstrated that the left sylvian fissure is consistently longer and more horizontally placed, suggesting that there is more cortex at the left temporal-parietal junction than on the right. The most suggestive cortical asymmetry to explain language dominance has been the demonstration by Geschwind and Levitsky (1968) of an asymmetry in the size of the planum temporale (the portion of the auditory association cortex lying on the superior surface of the temporal lobe), with the left planum significantly larger in a majority of brains. This subtle but dramatic asymmetry has been confirmed by a number of other investigators (Campain and Minckler, 1976; Chi, Dooling and Gilles, 1977). The importance of the left auditory association cortex in the aphasia syndromes, particularly Wernicke aphasia, implies a key role for this anatomical asymmetry in the lateral dominance of language.

Together, these observations indicate significant (albeit subtle) differences between the two hemispheres that appear to underlie the unilateral specialization of cerebral function in the human. That the human brain has tendencies to lateralize function (unilateral dominance) appears undeniable; whether the anatomical differences noted are adequate, or even correct explanations, or that other as yet undiscovered asymmetries will be of greater importance can only be settled by future investigations.

Exceptions to Language Dominance

While the fact of unilateral hemispheric dominance for language has been convincingly demonstrated, there are exceptions which deserve comment. One exception, the inconsistency of hemispheric dominance among the nonright-handed has already been mentioned. This group comprises the largest and often the most misleading number of exceptions. Several additional sources of noncompliance deserve mention as they can also be misleading.

As noted in Chapter 1, children do not have strongly lateralized language dominance. The exact age at which one hemisphere takes on this specialized function is unknown and probably undeterminable, but it is generally accepted that young children have an equipotentiality of hemispheric specialization (i.e. either hemisphere can develop language competency) (Zangwill, 1960). Clinical observations indicate that the hemispheric equipotentiality decreases with advancing age; either hemisphere can assume language function up to the age of puberty, probably through the teens and possibly for a number of years thereafter. The younger the patient, the less consistent the unilateral location of language dominance appears to be and, parenthetically, the better the prognosis for improvement after onset of aphasia.

A second suggested exception deserves close scrutiny. For many years investigators have been reporting cases of crossed aphasia, right-handed individuals who become aphasic following right-hemisphere damage. Most such reports describe individual cases; the frequency of crossed aphasia is difficult to gauge, probably no greater than 1 case in 300 or 400 right-handed aphasics. In view of the possibility that a number of right handers have some degree of mixed dominance, this number appears surprisingly small. In actuality, even this number may be inflated. In a study of reported cases of crossed aphasia, Boller (1973) noted than an inordinately large percentage (77 percent) were victims of either trauma or tumor involving the right hemisphere. As noted in Chapter 3, both of these sources of aphasia tend to disturb hemispheric function bilaterally. It appears quite possible that the aphasia in many of the reported cases was not crossed at all. None of the cases in the Boston Veterans Administration Hospital series (Table 13-1) had an unexplained crossed aphasia. It appears likely that crossed aphasia may be even less common than the low frequency generally suggested.

In summary, even the exceptions to the observation of unilateral hemispheric language dominance do not contradict the finding. The tendency for the left hemisphere to serve as the language master (in the right-handed individual) is tremendous and must be accepted as a clinical-neuroanatomical landmark of significance.

15

Localization of Language Functions

With the solid establishment of one clinical-neuroanatomical correlation of language function, the dominance of the left hemisphere, it is reasonable to look for additional correlations. Historically it was the demonstration of functional-anatomical correlations that produced the early surge of interest in aphasia. Several language functions have long been thought to have predictable anatomical localizations and several others have less accepted but still suggestive relationships with specific neuroanatomic localizations. Some of these correlations will be discussed in this chapter. In must be remembered that the language functions discussed have been and remain artificial, not physiological, and that future correlations may focus on totally different language activities. Nonetheless, useful information can be gained by study of the anatomical localizations of a number of language functions.

CONVERSATIONAL SPEECH

Without question, most observers consider the most striking feature of aphasia to be the abnormality of conversational (spontaneous) speech. Both the patient and the observers are painfully aware of the problems of verbal output. While a qualitative difference in aphasic output abnormalities has been recognized for many years, correlation of this functional difference with neuroanatomical localization is still not widely acknowledged. As early as 1868 Hughlings Jackson (1932) reported that his aphasic patients could be divided into two classes, those with no words and those who had plenty of words but make mistakes, a succinct and accurate differentiation. Wernicke (1874, 1908) utilized the terms *fluent* and *nonfluent* to describe the obvious difference in aphasic output and suggested an anatomical correlation for the two outputs. While misleading, the terms fluent and nonfluent have remained in the literature and a number of formal studies performed in recent years have reemphasized the significance of the dichotomy in aphasic verbal output.

The differentiating features of fluent and nonfluent output have been outlined in Chapter 4. Utilizing the clinical descriptions outlined, aphasic patients have been divided into those with primarily fluent and those with primarily nonfluent output. In the author's study (1967) the conversational language of

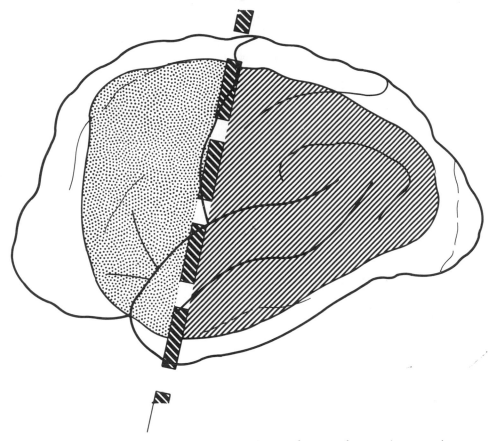

Figure 15-1. *Lateral view of left hemisphere indicating the anterior-posterior split separating nonfluent from fluent aphasic output.*

100 stable aphasics (at least one month post onset) was evaluated and approximately two out of three were readily placed in either a fluent or nonfluent category. Each patient had a radioactive isotope brain scan and the type of output, fluent or nonfluent, was correlated with the location of the lesion as demonstrated by the brain scan. The results were almost absolute. Patients classed as nonfluent had a locus of pathology anterior to Rolando's fissure (central sulcus) while those considered fluent had pathology posterior to this demarcation. This demonstration was neither radical nor unexpected; in fact, it agrees entirely with the observations and predictions Wernicke published in 1874. For some reason, however, these findings have never been widely accepted, and until recently an anatomical correlation with types of aphasic output had been actively denied by many aphasiologists. Two large and careful replications of this study have been performed (Poeck, Kerschensteiner and Hartje, 1972; Wagenaar, Snow and Prins, 1975), both supporting the anterior-posterior dichotomy of the spontaneous verbal output in aphasia.

Some exceptions to the anterior-posterior correlation are important and deserve note. In the first place, not all aphasics can be classed as fluent or nonfluent. In the author's study, approximately one-third of the aphasics evaluated could not be placed in this division with confidence. Studies that have failed to corroborate the fluent-nonfluent dichotomy (Karis and Horenstein, 1976) have had even greater numbers of patients whose output defied placement in one or another division. Obviously, not all aphasic patients have a clean anterior or posterior lesion (and a fair number have multiple lesions which may include both anterior and posterior loci), and if the clinical-anatomical correlation is correct, the presence of a sizeable number of patients who do not fit the dichotomy should be anticipated.

Other exceptions are also clinically noteworthy. Almost all children who become acutely aphasic are nonfluent (often they are mute), and even with recovery, almost never does a child develop a fully fluent, paraphasic, jargon type of output. Thus the acquired aphasia of childhood does not fit into the fluent-nonfluent division. Similarly, it is usually difficult to classify the output of left-handed aphasics, most showing a mixed fluent-nonfluent picture. While some left-handed patients can be placed clearly in one or the other of the output categories, for most the distinction is unclear. Finally, many patients with freshly acquired aphasia show nonfluent characteristics at the outset; some aphasics with posterior lesions rapidly become fluent but others may be nonfluent for weeks before altering to a fluent output. Evaluation in the early stages of aphasia may, therefore, be misleading, but always in the direction of nonfluency.

Thus, while the fluent-nonfluent dichotomy does offer significant anatomical localizing information it may not be applicable to an individual case. Nonetheless, for the practicing physician the two types of aphasic output often provide readily available and eminently useful neuroanatomical localizing information. By simply monitoring the output of an aphasic patient, an anatomical localization on an anterior-posterior axis can be demonstrated in many cases. The anterior-posterior information augments the correlation information concerning lateralization (right-left) and the two correlations provide a solid foundation on which to place additional localizing information. If an anatomical correlation can be made from the quality of conversational output, can similar information be deduced from other language parameters? The remainder of this chapter will explore this possibility.

REPETITION OF SPOKEN LANGUAGE

The ability to repeat exactly what the examiner has said may not be the most salient of language functions but it is a key finding in the aphasia exam and is one that is often overlooked. Abnormalities of the ability to repeat have always been noted and carefully studied by Continental aphasiologists but have not been emphasized in the English language discussions until recent years. Jackson (1932), Head (1926), Nielsen (1936), Schuell (1957), Brain (1961) and Wepman (1961), either failed to recognize the significance of repetition or failed to emphasize it in their writings on aphasia. The ability or lack of ability to repeat are both important findings in aphasia with significant connotations for the clinician.

One recent classification of the aphasias (Benson and Geschwind, 1971) uses success or failure in the repetition act as a key for classifying aphasia, a concept that has been modified only slightly for the present volume. Three well-known varieties of aphasia feature abnormal repetition, Broca aphasia, Wernicke aphasia and conduction aphasia (see Ch. 7). In dramatic contrast are the varieties of aphasia in which repetition is normal or strikingly superior to other language functions such as the transcortical motor and transcortical sensory varieties and the combination called mixed transcortical aphasia (see Ch. 8).

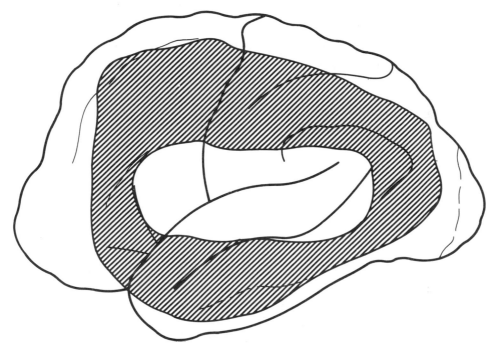

Figure 15-2. Lateral view of the left hemisphere indicating perisylvian area (*central clear*) where pathology is found if aphasic patient has repetition difficulty and borderzone area (*outer lined*) where pathology is suggested if aphasic patient can repeat adequately.

(Repeat Vs non repeat)

Correlating the types of aphasia in these two major subclasses with the location of the underlying pathology demonstrates an important distinction. The three types of aphasia with abnormal repetition all have pathology located in the immediate perisylvian region. Broca aphasia typically indicates structural damage in the posterior-inferior frontal lobe, Wernicke aphasia in the posterior-superior temporal region and conduction aphasia most often follows damage somewhere in the posterior perisylvian region, between the other two areas. In contrast, a distinct aphasia with preservation of the ability to repeat almost invariably indicates that the damage is located outside the immediate perisylvian area, somewhere in the borderzone area. Cases of transcortical motor aphasia usually indicate structural damage located anterior and/or superior to Broca's area. Transcortical sensory aphasia stems from damage in the parietal-temporal junction region posterior to Wernicke's area and the mixed transcortical syndrome points to fairly extensive borderzone (watershed) lesion(s) involving the cortex surrounding the perisylvian region. Thus monitoring the patient's ability to repeat can indicate localization of pathology into either the perisylvian or the arterial borderzone areas (see Fig. 15-2).

Not only is the differentiation between the perisylvian and the borderzone types of aphasia as determined by the ability to repeat a valid localizing feature, but it offers a practical diagnostic clue for the clinician. When vascular disease is the etiology, most aphasias with normal repetition are based on occlusive disease of the left internal carotid artery. Following acute occlusion of the carotid vessel, the limited arterial circulation available through the circle of Willis may be sufficient to perfuse only the immediate perisylvian cortex, allowing this area to remain viable but not providing sufficient oxygenated blood to maintain the borderzone tissues. In contrast, a CVA producing an aphasia with repetition disturbance is most likely based on thrombotic or embolic vascular problems with involvement of one or more of the branches of the middle cerebral artery. Thus, simply by testing repetition, valuable clinical findings in aphasia are available.

COMPREHENSION OF SPOKEN LANGUAGE

The ability to comprehend spoken language is routinely difficult to test and frequently misinterpreted (see Ch. 4). Comprehension is almost universally regarded as an all-or-none phenomenon: either the patient comprehends or he does not. This oversimplification of test interpretation causes many additional problems in an already difficult evaluation. Variations are rather obvious among the problems caused by comprehension difficulty but may not be easily demonstrated or categorized (particularly by pass-fail style examinations). Analysis of comprehension capability demands a great deal of care and thought and can provide valuable clinical insights as well as useful anatomical localizing data. For the present anatomical discussion, four distinctly different varieties of comprehension disturbance will be described. While they will be presented as totally separate entities, in actual practice there is almost always overlap of two or more of these problems, complicating but not completely obscuring the distinctions.

One disturbance of comprehension can be classed as a *receptive* problem. This aphasic patient shows severe disability in both comprehension and repetition of spoken language, but in sharp contrast he or she comprehends written language at a near normal level (this syndrome, called "pure word deafness" has been outlined in Ch. 13). Structural lesions in this disorder are most frequently located deep in the dominant temporal lobe, usually involving Heschl's gyrus and/or its afferent connections (see Fig. 15-3).

A second variety of comprehension disability is closely related to the first and can be called a *perceptive* problem. In this situation not only are comprehension and repetition of spoken language abnormal but a similar disability is found in the comprehension of written language (alexia). The degree of alexia roughly mirrors the severity of the auditory comprehension problem. Traditionally, this combination of clinical findings has been called Wernicke aphasia

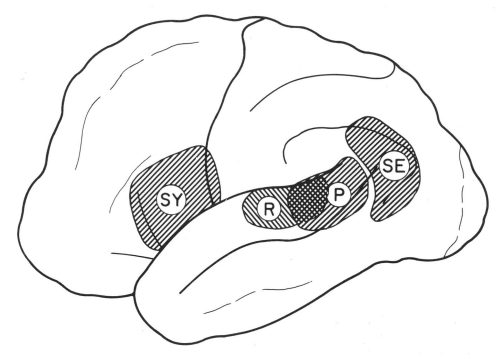

Figure 15-3. *Lateral view of left hemisphere indicating areas where four varieties of comprehension difficulty are likely to have pathology. Sy = anterior area associated with syntactic and sequencing problems, R = receptive area (actually subcortical) where pathology is often found in cases of pure word deafness, P = perceptive area (cortical surface) associated with Wernicke aphasia and SE = semantic area.*

and indicates pathology involving the cortex of the posterior-superior temporal area of the dominant hemisphere (Fig. 15-3). The locations of pathology underlying pure word deafness and Wernicke aphasia lie in close proximity, making mixtures of these syndromes so common as to be the rule. Nonetheless, pure cases of each type do occur and demonstrate a clear clinical distinction in comprehension disability that can be correlated with a small but significant difference in the location of pathology.

A third variety of comprehension disturbance can be described as a *semantic* problem and is less common, at least in pure form, although occurring frequently in mixed states. The patient with a semantic comprehension disturbance has difficulty understanding both spoken and written language, but unlike the previous types this patient can repeat spoken language accurately. Semantic comprehension disturbance is frequently incomplete, the patient comprehending some general information from conversation but showing an inordinate problem in understanding specific words. The patient with this problem apparently receives and perceives the auditory signal adequately, as demonstrated by the accurate verbal repetition of what has been said, but has inordinate difficulty extracting meaning from the verbal signals. While the location of the lesion in cases of semantic comprehension disturbance is less well defined and considerably more controversial, many investigators implicate the parietal-temporal borderzone area, the angular gyrus and its immediate connections in the posterior-inferior temporal cortex (see Fig. 15-3). Mixtures of semantic comprehension disturbance with one or both of the previously described types are extremely frequent, but again pure cases can be seen in clinical practice.

Finally, a fourth and totally different type of comprehension disturbance can be demonstrated. These aphasic patients comprehend individual words without difficulty but misunderstand sentence-length material. While this phenomenon is common and relatively easy to demonstrate, investigation of the defect in comprehension has proved difficult, leading to a number of possible explanations. One suggestion is that the patient cannot maintain language material in an accurate sequence (Albert, 1972); another implies an abnormality in the ability to comprehend syntactic or relational language structures (Zurif, Caramazza and Myerson, 1972; Samuels and Benson, 1979). When this is the only comprehension difficulty noted in an aphasic patient, the underlying pathology usually involves the dominant frontal lobe (in other words, Broca's area or surrounding structures). Pathology in the posterior language areas, however, can also interfere with both the handling of sequences and the comprehension of relational, grammatical structures; in this situation, however, the other comprehension deficits (described above) are also present. When comprehension problems are limited to the deciphering of material dependent upon multiple sequential bits of information or the relationship established by syntactic structures (articles, conjunctions, prepositions), frontal language area pathology is usually present. Figure 15-3 schematically illustrates the anterior language area thought to be abnormal when this type of comprehension disturbance occurs in a pure state.

The four varieties of comprehension defect described above are both operationally and anatomically separable, rather clearly demonstrating that attempts to deal with comprehension deficit as a unitary activity are misleading. It must be conceded, however, that a number of other approaches to comprehension defect could be suggested (e.g. disturbance based on specific categories such as colors or body parts, modalities such as visual recognition and word frequency). Future studies of language comprehension must recognize that it is not an all-or-none phenomenon and that anatomical correlations with the varieties of comprehension defect are probable.

WORD-FINDING DISABILITY

Anomia, a difficulty in finding or producing the correct word, is almost universally present in aphasia but has proved difficult to localize and there is a strong tendency to view naming difficulty as an all-or-none phenomenon. Even casual observation reveals distinct variations in naming disorders and many correlations of the different types of anomia with different subdivisions of naming have been presented, including such diverse attributes as animate-inanimate (Nielsen, 1940), developmental acquisition (Rochford and Williams, 1962), word frequency (Rochford and Williams, 1965), picturability (Goodglass, Barton and Kaplan, 1968) and operativity (Gardner, 1973). The variations to be described here fit none of these categorizations; rather, they reflect differences in word-finding problems noted in clinical aphasia examinations (Luria, 1966; Benson, 1979). Five distinct varieties of aphasic anomia will be described and it is recognized that more exist. Thus anomia is a prominent finding in a number of nonaphasic mental conditions such as dementia, confusional state, etc. As these conditions do not provide anatomical correlation information they will be excluded; the types of anomia to be discussed here all occur as part of an aphasic syndrome. The types of aphasic anomia outlined here are also discussed in detail elsewhere, with more extensive descriptions of varieties, suggestions for testing word-finding, case studies, anatomical correlations and a postulation of the neuroanatomy underlying the act of finding a word (Benson, 1979).

Word Production Anomia

This type of anomia refers to a difficulty in which the patient cannot produce the correct word even when appearing to know what is wanted. On confrontation-naming the patient fails to produce many words unless aided by prompting. The primary defect appears to be a problem in initiating articulation, although defective articulation and inability to name (despite extensive prompting) are often intermixed. A second, quite different problem in word-production occurs when the patient's output is so contaminated by paraphasia (usually phonemic substitutions or neologisms) that the required word is not presented. Often the number of syllables and the inflection are correct but the name produced is totally incorrect because of phoneme substitution. Both of these types of anomia feature inability to produce the correct word rather than lack of knowledge of the desired word. In most cases of word-production anomia, the pathology is located anteriorly, either involving the motor speech area of the left frontal lobe (such as Broca aphasia) causing articulatory initiation problems, or the pathways leading to Broca's area (for instance, conduction aphasia) producing excessive literal paraphasia. Figure 15-4 illustrates the areas involved in word production anomia.

Word Selection (Word Dictionary) Anomia

In some aphasic individuals the anomia appears to be based on an inability to select (find) the appropriate word. When asked to name an object the patient may deny remembering the name but can offer an adequate functional description of the item. Phonemic cues are rarely helpful to these patients, even when the cue includes most of the name of the object. In contrast, however, the patient can choose the correct item from an array of objects when the name is given by the examiner. Difficulty in entry to, or use of, a hypothetical lexical repository (the so-called word dictionary) is suggested as the cause (Katz and Foder, 1964; Brown, 1972). Pathology in these cases of "pure" anomia is usually located either in the posterior portion of the second temporal gyrus or in Brodmann's area 37, the temporal-occipital junction area of the dominant hemisphere (see Fig. 15-4). These two regions are contiguous and may be functionally related; at present there is too little material with discretely localized pathology to allow a statement separating or combining their function. However, a type of anomia featuring isolated word-selection problems does exist and has pathology rather consistently present in the posterior-inferior temporal region.

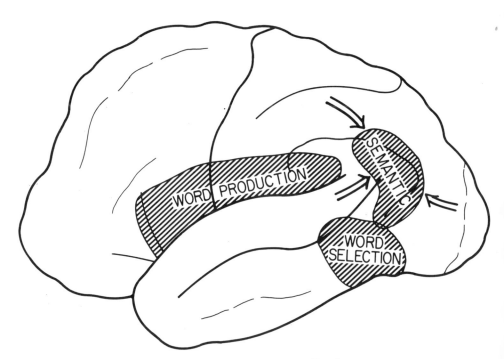

Figure 15-4. *Lateral view of left hemisphere indicating separate areas associated with varieties of anomia. The arrows diagrammatically indicate pathology interfering with transmission of sensory material to the language area.*

Semantic Anomia

This is a third distinct type of anomia. The patient with this problem also fails to present words upon confrontation-testing and will not accept cues, but unlike patients with word-selection anomia, patients with this variety cannot select the correct item from an array when the name is offered. The patient with semantic anomia appears to have lost (or forgotten) the symbolic meaning of the word (the word no longer represents the object). This phenomenon, under different names, has been discussed at length by Goldstein (1924), Head (1926) and Luria (1966). The location of pathology in semantic anomia is less exactly known but the area of the dominant angular gyrus is most often suggested (see Fig. 15-4). Again, the close proximity of the angular gyrus to the cortical area implicated in word-selection anomia portends frequent mixtures of the two types of word-finding difficulty, a clinical truism. Both varieties are seen in "pure" state, however, and represent an additional anatomical-pathological correlation.

Category-Specific and Modality-Specific Anomia

In addition to the three varieties of anomia mentioned above, two others deserve attention. Modality-specific anomia refers to a failure to name through a single modality of sensory input. Thus a patient with visual agnosia cannot name an object on visual confrontation but succeeds when allowed to palpate it. Category-specific anomia, on the other hand, refers to an inability to produce names from one category in contrast to other categories which are named adequately. Color anomia is the best-recognized example. While a number of varieties of modality-specific and category-specific anomia have been reported, they are seen infrequently in clinical practice and most have been reported only as individual case studies. The common feature to these two anomias is structural involvement of either a primary sensory area (such as the primary visual cortex) or pathways connecting such an area to the language area. In Figure 15-4 the locus of pathology underlying modality and category specific types of anomia is diagrammatically represented only by arrows in the posterior portion of the hemisphere, indicating connections between the primary sensory areas and angular gyrus.

While almost routinely intermixed, it is obvious from the short descriptive sketches that clinical variations in word-finding disturbance are observed by the clinician. To a considerable extent these variations of anomia can be correlated with the neuroanatomical site of pathology described. Improved language-testing techniques and advanced means of anatomical localization promise considerably better correlations in the future. Certainly anomia is not a unitary disturbance and some of the differences reflect the neuroanatomical site of pathology.

READING DISTURBANCES

As noted in Chapter 11, two varieties of reading disability (alexia) with different neuroanatomical loci of pathology have been recognized for many years and represent one of the more widely accepted clinical-anatomical correlations of language function. Recent observations have suggested a third common but clearly distinct variety of alexia with a separate neuroanatomical locus of pathology. The first two types of alexia were clearly outlined by Dejerine (1891 and 1892) and have been given a variety of names over the years. In this volume they are termed *occipital alexia* and *parietal-temporal alexia,* names that fully imply the anatomical correlation. The third variety, proposed recently, has been called *frontal alexia.* Clinical descriptions of these three types of alexia have been presented in detail in Chapter 11 and need not be repeated. Suffice it to say that there are many clinical points allowing differentiation of the three types of alexia and that correlation with the anatomical locus of pathology is readily established. Figure 15-5 graphically illustrates the anatomical separation of the regions implicated in the three varieties of aphasia.

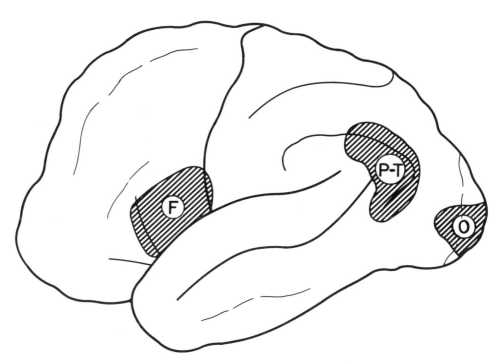

Figure 15-5. *Lateral view of the left hemisphere indicating suspected centers of pathology in the three major varieties of alexia. The extent of these areas is unknown but probably considerably greater than indicated on the diagram.*

AGRAPHIA

Disturbances in writing ability are extremely common in aphasia but have defied clinical differentiation and exact anatomical correlation. As discussed in

Chapter 12, many characteristics of agraphia can be separated out and at least some appear to have implications for anatomical localization. Nonetheless, the evidence supporting separate clinical-anatomical correlations for agraphia is too scanty at present to warrant localization statements other than the speculative dominant anterior, dominant posterior and nondominant separation suggested in Chapter 12. That significant variations in agraphia exist appears very likely, and experience suggests that the variations should reflect a neuroanatomical correlation. To date, however, the necessary clinical studies to separate varieties of agraphia have not been performed and specific anatomical correlations cannot be offered.

SUMMARY

Certain of the language functions described in Chapters 14 and 15 appear to have strong associations with specific neuroanatomical locations, and as such they offer valuable information for the diagnostician. This is particularly true of the lateralization of language function to the left hemisphere, the anatomical correlations of the fluent and nonfluent outputs and the ability to repeat. These distinctive variations in abnormal language features can be used with considerable assurance for the localization of cerebral pathology.

The other language functions mentioned above are not so readily utilized for anatomical localization; not only does their differentiation demand a considerable degree of clinical sophistication but the anatomical correlates are considerably more complex than the simple dichotomies of the other features. Nonetheless, clinical observation strongly suggests that the clinical-anatomical correlations described in this chapter are reliable and offer useful information, not only to the clinician but also to the student of language.

Many of the correlations described here have only recently been suggested. Improvement in language-testing skills and/or the use of a totally different set of functions may offer opportunities for better correlations in the future. And, of course, future technical advances in neuroanatomical localization in the living aphasic patient should also enhance the accuracy of the correlations. Clinical-anatomical correlation information of the type described here may be used by the clinician to augment data obtained by study of the aphasic syndromes, and in addition promises new avenues for language research. The "centers" for a given language function were discredited, but the concept of a "general" language function without anatomical correlation is just an untenable. Quite possibly further investigation of the anatomical structures underlying language functions along the lines outlined in this chapter will offer a better base for understanding language.

16

Associated Neurobehavioral Problems

Despite the implications provided by most discussions of language disorder, aphasia almost *never* occurs as an isolated neurobehavioral finding. As noted in Chapter 15, language functions are performed in many areas of the brain involving a sizeable portion of the left hemisphere, areas not only significant for language but essential for other behavioral activities. Damage that produces aphasia is likely to cause other forms of behavioral malfunction. Almost every individual with aphasia shows some additional neurobehavioral problem and these complicate the understanding of aphasia. A great deal of accumulated research data, both past and current, is contaminated by unrecognized neurobehavioral complications.

Many of the neurobehavioral complications of aphasia are poorly understood. Even well-trained clinicians have comparatively little experience recognizing, or dealing with, some of the nonverbal behavioral disturbances, and when unrecognized these complications interfere with both diagnosis and therapy. Some neurobehavioral disturbances totally negate aphasia therapy efforts and careful multidisciplinary evaluation should be performed on aphasics to establish candidacy for aphasia rehabilitation. Unfortunately, evaluations of this type are available in very few institutions at present. More clinicians with interest and training in the neurological aspects of behavior are needed before this demand can be met.

This chapter will present a compilation of neurobehavioral problems that are frequently associated with aphasia. The list is far from complete. Many of the neurobehavioral abnormalities produced by brain damage are poorly understood and the entire field deserves additional attention. The descriptions presented here are of necessity only sketches, and if the clinician wishes additional knowledge on the topic, selected areas of current literature must be reviewed. Among the recommended presentations are such books as *Behavioral Neurology* (Pincus and Tucker, 1974), *Psychiatric Aspects of Neurologic Disease* (Benson and Blumer, 1975) and *Organic Psychiatry* (Lishman, 1978), plus a growing number of articles in leading neurology, psychiatry and neuropsychology journals.

HEMIPLEGIA

Unilateral motor disturbance is so common in aphasia that, at least in its more gross forms, it is not overlooked. Approximately 80 percent of nonfluent aphasics show some degree of unilateral motor paralysis and about 20 percent of fluent aphasics also show significant motor disturbance (Howes and Geschwind, 1964). The degree of the motor problem is variable, ranging from a total right hemiplegia with almost no ability to move the right side to subtle disturbances limited to fine digital movements. Unilateral motor disturbance is present in many more aphasic patients than usually recognized, and the more subtle forms may cause considerable disability and are a fertile source of mis-diagnosis (often referred to as a malingering, hysterical reaction or some other psychologic explanation for the inept performance). Therapy is available for the motor disturbances and the reader is referred to some of the current guides for the rehabilitation of stroke (Lehman, DeLateur and Fowler, 1975; Sahs and Hartman, 1976) for additional details. Rehabilitation measures aimed at improv-ing motor activities play a significant role in aphasia therapy. The aphasic patient who can operate a wheel chair is a far better therapy candidate than one confined to bed. Successful ambulation often appears to be accompanied or followed by improvements in language retraining. While no absolute correla-tions of the results of physical rehabilitation and aphasia rehabilitation are available, active physical rehabilitation measures are obviously important for the aphasic patient with a unilateral motor disturbance.

PSEUDOBULBAR PALSY

This clinical syndrome can be traced to a variety of etiologies, is known by a number of terms (*spastic bulbar palsy, supranuclear bulbar palsy, pseudobul-bar palsy*) and is far more common as a complication of aphasia than generally recognized. The syndrome results when disease process (stroke, trauma, neo-plasm, degeneration) involves the upper motor neuron system bilaterally, and it gets its name by producing a false impression of lower brain stem (bulbar) malfunction.

Symptoms of pseudobulbar palsy are variable but fall into three major categories. First, there is evidence of motor disability, including bilateral hemiparesis, incontinence and bradykinesia. The degree of paresis may be slight, however, obscuring the diagnosis. A second group of symptoms is characterized by bulbar malfunction including dysphagia, drooling, choking, hoarseness, hypophonia, expressionless facies and decreased blinking. The third group, considered the most characteristic by many, features abnormal emotional expression. Best described as a lability of emotional expression, many pseudobulbar patients produce an excessive emotional response to an appropriate stimulus (Lieberman and Benson, 1977). Thus a situation in which mild unhappiness might be appropriate (i.e. mention of home or family) generates paroxysms of grief with sobbing, crying, moaning, facial distortions and the production of real tears. Such outbursts can be physically draining. Uncontrollable laughter can result from mildly happy stimuli in a similar manner and a shift from a happy to a sad expression of affect (or vice versa) may occur without additional stimulation. If questioned following cessation of the outburst, the patient often denies any emotional feeling except embarrassment caused by the inability to control the emotional expression. Clinically, excessive laughter appears to be more frequent in younger pseudobulbar patients while sadness and crying are more often seen in the older patient. The lability of emotional expression appears to be a loss of the ability to inhibit the emotional responses, rather than true emotional lability.

As already noted, the pseudobulbar state is a product of bilateral brain insult and many patients with this disorder suffer deteriorated mental functions. Such degeneration is not universal, however, and some patients retain normal or near-normal intellectual capacity beneath their grotesque physical and affective appearance. The full symptom picture may not be present. Some patients with severe bilateral motor problems have little emotional abnormality, others have severe problems controlling emotional expression but show little motor disability or bulbar symptomatology.

The neuroanatomical locus of pathological involvement varies from motor cortex to upper brain stem, centering at the internal capsule level; while always bilateral, the degree and level of involvement may be different in the two hemispheres. Currently there is disagreement as to whether pseudobulbar palsy results from pyramidal or extrapyramidal motor involvement, or both. While some cases are clearly spastic, many pure extrapyramidal disorders produce pseudobulbar features (e.g. parkinsonism).

For the aphasic, pseudobulbar palsy is a serious complication. The bulbar paresis interferes with phonation and the emotional overflow severely distorts spontaneous verbalization. Language therapy is difficult, but if intellectual deterioration is not too severe, a trial of individual therapy may prove beneficial.

HEMISENSORY LOSS

Sensory loss is often less obvious in the aphasic but is probably at least as common as motor disturbance. Inasmuch as sensory changes are not visible and many aphasics are unable to verbalize the alteration, sensory disturbance is frequently overlooked. Even when the patient has sufficient output, the complaint may be of clumsiness or heaviness in the limbs, misleading the examiner. Observations of subtle changes, such as a tendency for disuse of a limb despite absence of paralysis or an unexplained clumsiness of a fully powered limb, should suggest hemisensory loss. Demonstration of sensory alteration often proves frustratingly difficult because of the patient's inability to understand the tasks or to articulate a response to the stimulus. Perseverative or overly cooperative responses are common, and generally useless. Even with careful, intuitive testing, sensory problems often remain undiscovered. Therapy for sensory disorder is far less positive, but some treatments, particularly those emphasizing digital activities, appear helpful. Demonstration of the problem to the patient and attempts to teach compensatory maneuvers also may be of value.

VISUAL FIELD DEFECT

Visual field defects are common in individuals with aphasia, particularly those whose pathology is posterior. The visual field defect may be of little consequence to the aphasia or its rehabilitation, but in one correlative study the presence of sensory loss, including visual field defect, presaged a poor prognosis (Smith, 1972). Many neuropsychological studies have used the presence or absence of visual field defects as a comparison point and consistently demonstrate that patients with visual field defects have more problems handling sensory input than brain-damaged individuals with full visual fields (DeRenzi, Faglioni and Scotti, 1970; Chedru, Leblanc and Lhermitte, 1973). Although few studies to date have formally separated visual field defect from unilateral inattention, the presence or absence of neglect (see next section) appears to be of greater consequence. Nonetheless, the presence of a quadrantic or full half-field visual defect may interfere with language function, and patients with these defects appear to have a poorer prognosis for aphasia rehabilitation.

UNILATERAL INATTENTION

A number of clinically separable problems are presently recognized, ranging from 1) a tendency to neglect one side to 2) unconcern about all or part of the body on one side through 3) unawareness of all but major stimuli to one side to 4) anosagnosia (outright denial of any problems involving the entire side of the body) (Critchley, 1953; Benson and Geschwind, 1975). Most reports suggest that all aspects of unilateral inattention occur most often to patients with right hemisphere pathology (Brain, 1945; Hecaen, 1962; Gainotti, Messerli and Tissot, 1972; Oxbury, Campbell and Oxbury, 1974). It should be noted, however, that neglect of the right side is not at all uncommon in left-hemisphere damaged patients and can complicate aphasia rehabilitation. Full anosagnosia is considerably less common following left hemisphere than right hemisphere damage, possibly because the severely aphasic patient cannot readily express denial of bodily problems. One recent study of over 100 acute stroke cases demonstrated some evidence of anosagnosic phenomena in 87 percent with left paresis (right hemisphere damage) while only about 24 percent of those with right hemiplegia had an abnormal attitude towards their paralysis (Cutting, 1978). However, over half of the severe right hemiplegics were too aphasic to either admit or deny their paresis, and if all aphasics were considered to hold an abnormal attitude, the number of left-hemisphere damaged patients in this group climbs to 81 percent. The possibility that severe unilateral inattention follows insult to either hemisphere cannot be dismissed. The clinician, however, must rely on observations rather than verbalizations for evidence suggesting neglect or inattention in aphasic individuals. If the patient tends to ignore persons on his right side, if there is a tendency to draw or to write on the left hand side of the paper only, if close attention is paid to stimuli on the left but much stronger stimuli are needed to get attention on the right, then a significant unilateral inattention must be suspected. The stimuli used for testing may be visual, auditory or somesthetic, and frequently the patient with inattention in one modality will have problems in all three. A number of theories as to the cause of unilateral inattention have been raised (DeRenzi, Faglioni and Scotti, 1970; Gainotti, Messerli and Tissot, 1972; Heilman, Watson and Schulman, 1974; Watson and Heilman, 1978), all of which may be partially correct, but the explanations remain both hypothetical and controversial. It is sufficient to state that unilateral inattention may be an important finding in patients with aphasia, may adversely affect therapy and demands consideration by both clinician and language therapist.

DISORDERS OF EXTRAOCULAR MOVEMENT

True extraocular motor palsies are not common as complications of aphasia. In fact, when a patient with acute aphasia shows an extraocular motor problem, the possibility that it is a congenital squint ranks high. Conjugate eye movement difficulty, on the other hand, is fairly common, particularly in the early course of aphasia. Difficulty in moving the eyes laterally (gaze paresis) may be seen in patients with acute lesions involving either frontal or parietal-occipital association cortex. Gaze paresis is analogous to paralysis of limb movement. Thus, weakness of limb movements on the right is often accompanied by weakness of conjugate gaze to the right. Lateral eye movements should be tested in two ways, the ability to move the eyes on command ("look to your right") and the ability to follow a moving object from side to side. Not infrequently there is a dissociation of gaze paresis, one function being fully preserved while unilateral gaze paresis is demonstrated with the other. The dissociation has considerable localizing value. Loss of conjugate eye movement to command indicates frontal eye field (Brodmann area 8) pathology whereas a similar loss to reflex movement (following) is seen with parietal-occipital eye field (area 18 & 19) damage. There is a strong tendency for conjugate deviation to be transient, however. While mild degrees of gaze palsy may persist, they characteristically become difficult to demonstrate early in the course of recovery. Careful testing may demonstrate some evidence of weakness of unilateral gaze toward the right (Holmes, 1918) and the possibility that this may affect the ability to read has been suggested (see Ch. 11).

SEIZURES, EPILEPSY

Epileptic seizures are a complication of consequence in the aphasic patient. Both general and partial (motor or sensory) seizures may occur, dependent upon the site of pathology. The frequency of seizures complicating aphasia is difficult to ascertain. It has been suggested that approximately 25 percent of patients suffering a cerebral-vascular accident develop seizures and that cerebral vascular accidents are the most common cause of first seizure in persons over the age of 60 (Adams and Victor, 1977). Our experience in managing sizeable numbers of aphasic patients suggests that these figures may be high, but there can be little doubt that the etiology of the aphasia is the key to whether seizures will occur. Tumors, cerebral trauma and neurosurgical procedures commonly lead to seizures. Some types of cerebral vascular accidents, particularly emboli, are more liable to cause seizure activity and seizures are most common when the cortex is damaged. Often there is a prolonged period (ranging from months to a year or more) between the onset of aphasia and the first seizure, invariably raising a question as to the relationship of the two events and often requiring a repeat neurodiagnostic evaluation. Most seizures in aphasic patients are controlled adequately by standard medication regimes, but anticonvulsant medications are potent, and by themselves can produce significant neurobehavioral side effects. Both the seizures and their treatment add to the problems of the aphasic patient.

MUTISM, HYPOPHONIA

The presence of abnormal voice volume is of considerable importance as a complicating factor and occurs with sufficient frequency to warrant attention. Neither hypophonia nor mutism (total lack of voice) is a symptom of aphasia and both occur most frequently in nonaphasic disorders. On the other hand, it cannot be said that an abnormality of vocalization precludes aphasia. The two conditions frequently coexist, at least temporarily. The most common cause of hypophonia is local inflammation of the larynx, often producing total mutism (laryngitis). Other peripheral sources of hypophonia include damage to the recurrent laryngeal nerve, nodules or polyps of the larynx and carcinoma of the larynx. While none are casually associated with aphasia, each deserves consideration. Aphasic patients can, and do, develop primary laryngeal pathology which is easily overlooked in the presence of major language deficiencies, a fertile source of error. In addition, pathology involving a number of cerebral areas can produce hypophonia. These include:

1. Broca's area itself where acute lesions may produce a transient mutism (see description of aphemia, Ch. 13);

2. dominant hemisphere supplementary motor area (Schwab, 1926; Penfield and Roberts, 1959);

3. the reticular substance of the mesencephalon where pathology can pro-

duce akinetic mutism but more commonly causes a degree of hypophonia (Segarra, 1970; Botez and Barbeau, 1971);

4. thalamus, particularly in cases of parkinsonism that have undergone thalamotomy (Riklan and Levita, 1970; Brown, 1974);

5. bilateral cerebral pathology, particularly when it affects the cortical and/or subcortical motor structures or pathways producing pseudobulbar palsy.

It is essential that the clinician investigate the cause of mutism or hypophonia in aphasic patients, and when possible treat the appropriate disorder. As a complication to aphasia, decreased vocalization interferes significantly with language therapy and recovery.

DYSARTHRIA

Dysarthria is best described as a group of speech disorders based on impaired motor control of the speech musculature. By tradition dysarthria refers only to those speech problems caused by neurologic dysfunction. While common in aphasia, dysarthria is not present in all aphasic syndromes and many dysarthric disorders have no language disturbance component. Many aphasiologists consider dysarthria separately, a complication of aphasia which indicates involvement of brain areas other than those subserving language. Others debate this point suggesting cortical sources of dysarthria that can be part of an aphasic syndrome (Trost and Canter, 1974). Dysarthria is present in many (but not all) cases of anterior aphasia but is relatively rare in posterior aphasia. The motor speech disorder accompanying the anterior aphasia syndromes has been called *cortical dysarthria, spastic dysarthria, verbal apraxia, cortical anarthria, efferent motor aphasia* and other names by various investigators, implying either a physiological or an anatomical correlation. Unfortunately, the descriptions provided for the speech abnormalities have been as broad and variable as the proposed names. Spastic problems predominate but other types of dysarthria do occur in aphasia and the combination of aphasia with dysarthria produces a challenging diagnostic puzzle.

Motor speech problems have proved extremely difficult to delineate and describe. In a massive and elegant study of dysarthria performed at the Mayo Clinic (Darley, Aronson and Brown, 1969, 1975) many speech parameters were monitored in a variety of neurological patients. Five major types of dysarthria were outlined:

1. Flaccid dysarthria (lower motor neuron paralysis) is characterized by hypernasality, breathy phonation and audible inspiration (stridor). This is the speech heard in bulbar paralysis (poliomyelitis, tumor, CVA) and myasthenia gravis.

2. Spastic dysarthria (upper motor neuron paralysis) is characterized by slow rate, low pitch, harsh quality, imprecise articulation and effortful phonation. This is the dysarthria heard most frequently with hemiplegia or pseudobulbar palsy.

3. Ataxic dysarthria (cerebellar) is characterized by irregularly broken articulation, equalization of stress on words and syllables, prolongation of phonemes and intervals and a slow, harsh, irregular tone and occurs in a number of cerebellar disorders.

4. Hypokinetic dysarthria (as seen in parkinsonism) features decreased variability (monotony) of pitch and loudness, hypophonia, reduced stress, imprecise articulation and inappropriate silences.

5. Hyperkinetic dysarthria has two variations. One has a rapid output with episodic hypernasality, harshness, breathiness and loudness, variable articulation, slow rate with prolonged intervals and equalized stress as seen in chorea. The second has a slow output with irregular articulation, variable harshness and breathiness and slowing due to prolongation of both phonemes and intervals as noted in dystonic speech.

Actually, even this outline fails to identify all recognized variations of dysarthria and all dysarthrias have proved extremely difficult to describe in words. In contrast, it is relatively easy for the observer to recognize and differentiate many of the more common dysarthric outputs (e.g. the dysarthria of parkinsonism from cerebellar dysarthria) when they are heard. Almost any type or combination of dysarthria can occur with aphasia, and for the uninitiated seriously confounds the language syndromes. Some of the dysarthrias are amenable to specific speech therapy techniques but not the techniques used for language therapy, another reason for careful diagnostic evaluation of the aphasia.

ACQUIRED STUTTERING

Stuttering is a deviation of speech characterized by irregular interruptions of the normal rhythm by involuntary repetition, prolongation or arrest of speech sounds. For some reason stuttering is easily overlooked in aphasia and has only rarely been noted as a significant complication. Several recent reports (Rosenbeck et al, 1978; Helm, Butler and Benson, 1978) suggest that acquired stuttering may be fairly common and may even have specific neuroanatomical correlations. Although appearing similar to the untrained ear, acquired stuttering and the far more common developmental stuttering have a number of demonstrable differences. Foremost is the observation that acquired stuttering occurs acutely (or possibly progressively in certain degenerative disorders) in an individual who has not previously stuttered. Helm, Butler and Benson (1978) reported five speech behaviors in acquired stuttering which differed from common features of the developmental variety. These included: 1) an absence of adaptation effect; 2) repetitions, prolongations and blocks were not restricted to the initial syllables; 3) stuttering involved grammatical as well as substantive words; 4) while the speaker might be annoyed by the stutter, there was no appearance of significant anxiety and 5) secondary symptomatology such as facial grimacing and fist clenching was rarely noted.

Many cases of acquired stuttering are transient, lasting up to eight weeks, but some have proved permanent. The study of Helm, Butler and Benson (1978) indicated that when stuttering was permanent, evidence of bilateral hemispheric involvement was always present. Transient acquired stuttering, on the other hand, followed left hemisphere insult, and in the few appropriately studied cases apparently depended upon involvement of multiple sites, either simultaneously (as with multiple emboli) or serially.

It has long been suggested that acquired stuttering is a motor speech complication and, as such, occurs almost exclusively with anterior (Broca) aphasia (Canter, 1971; Caplan, 1972). This appears untrue. The study of Helm, Butler and Benson demonstrated acquired stuttering in six aphasic patients, none of whom had a nonfluent output. Stuttering-like phenomena may occur in Broca aphasia (Trost, 1971) but not exclusively. At present there is no specific treatment for acquired stuttering; if present following unilateral hemispheric damage the outlook is promising, but when there is evidence of bilateral hemispheric damage the possibility of a permanent stutter appears high.

SCANNING SPEECH

For most neurologists, scanning speech is synonomous with multiple sclerosis (MS). Nystagmus, ataxia and scanning speech constitute "Charcot's triad," a classically recognized but overvalued syndrome of advanced multiple sclerosis. On this basis, scanning speech is widely but incorrectly attributed to cerebellar malfunction. Certainly this unusual verbal output does occur in some patients with MS, usually only at a far advanced stage, but MS is not the only pathology underlying scanning speech nor is it even the most common. And there is little evidence to support a cerebellar localization for scanning speech from any cause.

Scanning speech is characterized by a slow, deliberate, monotonous, segmented verbal output, usually presented as individual words. The output is grammatically and semantically intact but articulation is often, though not always, faulty, and of course the normal prosodic quality is entirely disrupted. These qualities, particularly the noteworthy dysprosody, suggest a nonfluent output and scanning speech is commonly mislabeled as anterior aphasia.

The most common cause of scanning speech in current medical practice appears to be trauma. It was clearly demonstrated in a superb study (Kremer, Russell and Smyth, 1947) of posttrauma patients who, following prolonged coma, showed third nerve dysfunction, an unusual combination of contralateral cerebellar ataxia and contralateral spasticity and scanning speech. The authors suggested a mesencephalic localization of pathology at a level just above the decussation of the brachium conjunctiva and supported their premise by demonstrating significantly enlarged aqueducts of Sylvius by air encephalography in three of their patients. A follow-up study (Boller et al, 1972) confirmed the enlargement of the sylvian aqueduct in many posttraumatic cases. Often overlooked in such studies is the appearance of scanning speech following mid-brain trauma. In the author's experience, trauma has been the most common and almost exclusive etiology of scanning speech. Of major import is the fact that scanning speech appears to indicate brain stem pathology, has no real association with aphasia and responds to speech therapy techniques, not aphasia therapy, points not recognized by many contemporary physicians and therapists.

PALILALIA

Palilalia is a unique, striking and comparatively rare speech disorder characterized by involuntary repetition of words or phrases during verbal output. In most instances, palilalia and aphasia are separate disorders but palilalia has been reported with both anterior and posterior aphasias with the combination producing confusing output disorders. Descriptions of palilalia date from the early 20th century, most frequently in individuals who had suffered encephalitis lethargica but also in cases demonstrating calcification of the basal ganglia. Most authorities have accepted palilalia as an indication of bilateral basal ganglia involvement (Brain, 1961). More recent experience suggests that this is not entirely true. We have seen classic palilalic output in individuals with basal ganglia pathology, but also in loose schizophrenics and even in cases of severe posterior aphasia. Efforts at treatment have been limited but recent experiences using a pacing board (Helm and Lieberman, 1977) show considerable promise.

CONFUSIONAL STATE

Confusional disturbances (often called delerium) are common, important and all too frequently overlooked problems that greatly complicate aphasia. If the confusional state is sufficiently pronounced it is obvious to the therapist and appropriate efforts can be made to correct the problem. In altogether too many cases, however, the findings are subtle or overlooked and the disorder causes great difficulty for the management of aphasic patients. Even the task of defining confusional states has proved difficult. In the broadest view, the inability to maintain a coherent line of thought has been considered the key property of a confusional state. Lines of thought are also abnormal in many of the disease processes with thought disorder (schizophrenia, depression, dementia) and are routinely difficult to recognize in the face of aphasia, so other criteria are necessary. Decreased digit span is often a sign but may be failed because of language disorder. Even observations of alertness and attention are made treacherous by problems of neglect, auditory comprehension disorder, reactive depression and other behavioral problems, particularly in the early stages of brain disorder when confusion is most common. There are many causes of confusional state, some based on structural pathology but most on functional abnormalities such as metabolic disturbance and drug intoxication. Confusional state must be ruled out in aphasia, particularly in the acute stages. Inasmuch as most of the causes of confusional state are treatable, considerable effort should be made to diagnose the underlying condition and to correct the problem. Obviously, aphasia therapy is ineffective for the patient in a confusional state and should await correction of the problem.

AMNESIA

Amnesia is a serious complicating factor of aphasia, one that is altogether too easy to overlook in the presence of language loss. In general terms, amnesia can be called a disturbance of memory, but it can be characterized more specifically as an inability to learn new material (Benson, 1978). To complicate matters, most formal tests of memory function, particularly tests of learning ability, are verbal and, therefore, have limited usefulness in an aphasic population. An additional complication stems from the fact that anomia superficially resembles a retrieval defect of memory (i.e. the patient cannot "remember" the name of an object or person). Actually, amnesia may affect the learning of names but most patients with true amnesia (such as Korsakoff's psychosis) have normal or near-normal spontaneous speech (they do not show the emptiness, circumlocution or pauses for word-finding seen in anomic aphasia) and can name on confrontation and produce normal word lists. Similarly, most patients with anomic aphasia demonstrate considerable ability to learn new material, i.e. learning the way about the ward, learning to recognize ward personnel and learning nonverbal means of communication. The two conditions, anomia and amnesia, are distinctly different and in most instances are readily distinguished by appropriate observations.

The pathology underlying amnesia varies with the etiology but the neuroanatomical locus usually includes structures deep in the medial aspect of the temporal lobe or in the diencephalon bilaterally, almost always involving portions of the inner core of the limbic system, the hippocampi, fornices and/or mammillary bodies (Brierley, 1966; Victor, Adams and Collins, 1971). Recent investigation, however, suggests that the key structures may be outside the limbic system. Involvement of the medial dorsal nucleus of the thalamus has been suggested by Victor, Adams and Collins (1971) and the temporal stem and postero-lateral temporal cortex have been implicated by Horel (1978). Among the recognized causes of amnesia, such entities as closed head trauma, herpes encephalitis, amnesic stroke and bitemporal tumor (or surgery) are likely to produce aphasia also. Pathological involvement in the temporal lobe may be sufficiently extensive to produce both amnesia and aphasia, an uncommon but not unknown combination. When present, amnesia is a serious complication of aphasia. The individual with a significantly compromised ability to learn is not a candidate for most current techniques of aphasia therapy and, to date, efforts made to devise therapy for patients with combined aphasia and amnesia have not been promising. Traditional therapy techniques prove frustrating and disappointing for both the patient and the therapist. Thus amnesia and aphasia present two major problems for the physician and the language therapist. One is the design of a reliable method for demonstrating amnesia in individuals with serious language deficits and the second is development of a means to treat aphasia successfully in the face of significantly impaired learning ability.

DEMENTIA

Dementia is another frequent and treacherous neurobehavioral complication of aphasia. Language disorder may occur as a sign of developing dementia, but, on the other hand, dementia may also result from the pathology that has produced an aphasia. The two conditions frequently coexist and in many instances are not specifically separable.

Dementia has always proved difficult to define (Lipowski, 1975; Wells, 1977). For present purposes the following operational definition can be suggested: *dementia* is an acquired impairment of intellectual capacity that includes abnormality in at least several of the following functions: 1) language, 2) memory, 3) visual-spatial ability, 4) cognitive ability and 5) personality.

Many different disorders can cause dementia (Haase, 1977), many of which can also produce aphasia. These include the Alzheimer or senile dementia syndrome, a degenerative brain disorder almost exclusively affecting the association cortex and hippocampus, in which a language disorder is a recognized feature that appears in the early stages. The aphasia of Alzheimer dementia is almost always limited to anomia and may not be a striking aspect. Nonetheless, a significant aphasic defect is a consistent finding. Another common cause of concurrent aphasia and dementia is the multi-infarct syndrome. When a patient suffers a number of separate vascular accidents, not only can an aphasia result but other neurobehavioral residua may be present in sufficient degree to warrant the diagnosis of dementia (Hachinski, Lassen and Marshall, 1974). A third source of combined aphasia and dementia is intracranial tumor, with or without corrective surgery. Tumors may produce widespread mental changes by increasing intracranial pressure, obstructing CSF outflow causing hydrocephalus, compressing major arterial feeders, and through either the necrosis of the tumor or a surgical decompression injuring brain tissue. Yet another common source of combined dementia and aphasia is intracranial trauma. When traumatic insult to the cortex and subcortical structures has been widespread, both language disorder and dementia may be present. Many other disorders such as intracranial infection, subarachnoid hemorrhage and metabolic-toxic state, affect cerebral tissues; and if sufficiently widespread can produce a combination of language disturbance and dementia, posing difficult diagnostic and therapeutic problems.

The differential diagnosis in patients with both dementia and aphasia may be obvious but also may be subtle and mysterious. Anomia is the most common variation of aphasia in cases of dementia but this relationship is not exclusive. The use of word lists (see Ch. 4) is a particularly useful diagnostic tool as most patients with dementing disorders perform badly when attempting to produce word lists. Most aphasics and many of the "normal aging" population present limited word lists, however, so that the test is not absolute for dementia. When a patient produces only a skimpy word list but does well on confrontation-naming tests, the possibility of a dementing disorder can be considered. The presence of other neurobehavioral disturbances such as a memory defect, constructional problems and alterations in personality are essential to establish a diagnosis of dementia. These may be difficult to demonstrate in the presence of aphasia. Unfortunately, most neuropsychological batteries are tilted heavily toward verbal testing and are of limited value in differentiating dementia and aphasia. Valuable insight can be gained from the nonverbal (performance) results but interpretation of these data demands experience. In particular, interpretation of nonverbal test results demands considerable background experience if used in an individual with aphasia; misinterpretation, almost always leading toward a diagnosis of dementia, is probable in the hands of the uninitiated.

The outlook when dementia and aphasia are combined depends entirely on the etiology. In general, though, when dementia complicates aphasia, the patient is a poor candidate for aphasia therapy. In this situation it is far better to seek the source of pathology, and if this is correctable the condition may be improved sufficiently for aphasia therapy to be beneficial.

GERSTMANN SYNDROME

The Gerstmann syndrome has been controversial almost since its introduction but continues to show up in discussions of aphasia and related neurobehavioral problems. The Gerstmann syndrome is said to be present when four findings occur together: right/left disorientation, finger agnosia, agraphia and acalculia (Gerstmann, 1931). The neurologic literature has long suggested that when all four symptoms are present, the pathology involves the left parietal region. In recent years, the existence of the Gerstmann syndrome has been disputed by a number of competent authorities (Benton, 1961, 1977; Heimburger, Demyer and Reitan, 1961; Critchley, 1966). They note that the full syndrome is rare in brain-damaged subjects and that the presence of any one or even several of the component signs fails to indicate dominant parietal pathology. One group (Poeck and Orgass, 1969) suggests that the presence of the Gerstmann syndrome merely indicates a subtle aphasia. This is not helpful; many cases of subtle and even nonsubtle aphasia do not have the features of the Gerstmann syndrome. Clinical experience supports Gerstmann's original observation; when all four symptoms are present, the probability that the patient has dominant parietal abnormality is considerable. It is true that several or even three of the components may be present when pathology is located elsewhere, but the actual syndrome demands all four components and, when demonstrated, has considerable value for localization. A syndrome featuring anomic aphasia, alexia with agraphia and the Gerstmann syndrome is fairly common, has been called the "angular gyrus syndrome" and represents as reliable localizing information as any syndrome in medicine.

VISUAL AGNOSIA

Visual agnosia is a distinctly uncommon (downright rare) disturbance in pure form, but it seems probable that less severe forms may be present in many posterior aphasics, hidden by the aphasia. Visual agnosia can be considered when the patient cannot recognize, on visual presentation, an object which he or she readily recognizes (and names) if allowed to feel, hear the sound of the object, etc. To warrant use of the term *visual agnosia,* the patient must have sufficient vision to see the object and sufficient language to use the name of the object in conversations, failing to name only on visual confrontation (Teuber, 1968; Rubens and Benson, 1971). Some refer to this disorder as a separate aphasia syndrome, optic aphasia (Freund, 1888; Lhermitte and Beauvois, 1973), but visual agnosia is used more commonly. Evidence suggests that pathology in cases of visual agnosia primarily involves the inferior portions of the occipital-temporal junction bilaterally (Lhermitte, Chain and Escourelle, 1972; Benson, Segarra and Albert, 1974; Levine, 1978). In the few relatively "pure" cases of visual agnosia described in the literature, associated findings have included hemianopsia (usually right-sided), prosopagnosia, constructional disturbance, alexia without agraphia, color-naming disturbance, amnesia and some degree of anomia. Less "pure" cases have even more evidence of posterior aphasia and more severe cognitive defects, masking the degree of visual agnosia. That visual agnosia is more common than can be demonstrated is almost a truism, and that it may be a significant complication in a fair number of cases of posterior aphasia deserves consideration.

AUDITORY AGNOSIA

Auditory agnosia is currently used to depict two distinctly different clinical conditions (Albert et al, 1972; Goldstein, 1974). One use indicates that auditory agnosia defines a condition in which the individual is unable to recognize *non-verbal* auditory stimuli, even though they can be heard; language sounds are readily understood by such a patient. In this definition, auditory agnosia is the obverse of pure word deafness. The second definition combines both conditions, an inability to interpret both verbal and nonverbal sounds even though the patient can hear the sounds (Oppenheimer and Newcombe, 1978). As pure word deafness has already been discussed (Ch. 13) this discussion will focus on the first use of auditory agnosia.

An isolated inability to recognize nonverbal sounds does exist and has been described clinically. These patients cannot recognize and identify sounds such as whistling, hand-clapping, a telephone ringing, or a dog barking, even though adequately responding to language sounds. The topic has been described in detail by several investigators (Spreen, Benton and Fincham, 1965; Vignolo, 1969) but considerable controversy remains concerning the site of the disturbance. Most often the right (nondominant) temporal area is thought to be involved (amnesia is frequently present). As such, auditory agnosia is not a complication of aphasia; often, however, it can be combined with or mistaken for a language problem and auditory agnosia may then be a complication of aphasia.

TACTILE AGNOSIA

A syndrome analogous to the visual and auditory agnosia disorders has recently been reported under the name *bilateral tactile aphasia* (Beauvois et al, 1978). In their remarkable case the patient was unable to name objects on palpating them but could give the names when they were visualized or heard. That lesser degrees of this problem may exist must be acknowledged, and if present could further complicate an aphasic problem.

APRAXIA

Apraxia is one of the most consistently misused terms in medical literature. Most of the types of apraxia currently described by medical and paramedical workers (e.g. verbal, constructional, dressing), represent fixed motor or visual-spatial disturbances and should not be defined by the term apraxia any more than a hemiplegia should. Despite the widespread misuse of apraxia to denote many types of motor performance failure, the presence of motor apraxia in individuals with aphasia is almost routinely overlooked.

Motor (better termed *ideomotor*) *apraxia,* defined as an inability to carry out on command an activity that can be performed spontaneously, is demonstrable in as many as 40 percent of aphasic patients when properly sought and is a complication of considerable importance in aphasia. Other types of apraxia, *glossokinetic apraxia* (essentially a tremor or clumsiness of limbs) and *ideational apraxia* (an inability to maintain the ideas necessary to carry out a complicated activity) occur less frequently but may also complicate aphasia. The latter two are much more difficult to define operationally or to demonstrate, however. Motor apraxia, on the other hand, is comparatively specific and easily demonstrated. Requests can be given for bucco-facial activities (whistling, coughing, sucking, blowing, winking, smiling), limb activities (making a fist, waving goodbye, saluting, shaking hands) and whole body actions (stand up, sit down, turn around, swing a golf club, kick a football). Failure to perform such acts on command when there is no paralysis, ataxia or comprehension defect suggests ideomotor apraxia. Even more subtle is the request to pretend the use of an object (comb, toothbrush, hammer); substitution of a body part for the object indicates ideomotor apraxia.

Apraxia of both bucco-facial and limb activities is seen frequently in Broca aphasia, transcortical motor aphasia and conduction aphasia. In some cases of aphemia a fairly restricted bucco-facial apraxia may be noted. Of paramount significance is the interference that apraxia produces in the testing of comprehension, particularly if comprehension is evaluated only through motor activities. For instance, ideomotor apraxia is a recognized but rarely emphasized source of failure on the Token Test (DeRenzi and Vignolo, 1962). The opposite is true also; comprehension defect must be ruled out before apraxia can be proved.

Many theories explaining the causes of apraxia are available in the current literature (Geschwind, 1965; Heilman, 1973; Hecaen and Albert, 1978), but demonstration of the basic disorder by physicians remains limited. Ideomotor apraxia is not only common but represents one of the most significant and frequently overlooked complications to both aphasia evaluation and aphasia therapy.

SUMMARY

The above descriptions, while sketchy, amply demonstrate that a great number of related abnormalities can and do seriously complicate aphasia. The presence of one or several neurobehavioral complications make both the evaluation and the treatment of aphasia difficult. It is strongly suggested that any patient being considered for aphasia therapy deserves a thorough evaluation for neurobehavioral complications by a team with skills in neurology, psychiatry, speech pathology and psychology before an arduous, difficult and expensive course of language rehabilitation is undertaken.

17

Psychiatric Aspects of Aphasia

Aphasia has obvious psychiatric implications, significant for both the aphasic and those caring for him or her. Despite a century of intense study, including a broad range of psychologic studies, and an entire method of treatment featuring psychogenic support (sympathy and understanding), relatively little attention has been given to the psychiatric problems which complicate aphasia. These problems often prove crucial to the ultimate outcome of the aphasic condition.

PSYCHOSOCIAL ASPECTS

The most important psychosocial factor affecting most individuals with aphasia stems from the sudden, unexpected and truly calamatous alteration of life style produced by the disorder. The overwhelming magnitude of this factor becomes obvious if we picture ourselves suddenly bereft of the ability to talk or to understand those about us. Language is so basic to human existence that its loss ranks with acute blindness or quadriplegia in psychic shock. In addition to the loss of language itself, changes occur in most of the stabilizing factors of personal existence such as employment status, social and family position, recreational opportunities and many others. The sudden, catastrophic onset of the aphasic condition by itself produces a massive psychic problem.

Among the many psychosocial problems plaguing the asphasic, alteration in economic status is a major concern for many. Aphasia often occurs at a stage when a person's earning capacity is near its prime, a time when the individual is comparatively independent and self-sufficient. This desirable status suddenly disappears, and, with growing awareness of their altered status, aphasics realize that their economic independence is permanently lost, a matter of deep concern.

Coupled with the change in economic status but entirely independent is a similar alteration in the aphasic's position in society. By the time aphasia occurs in most individuals, they have established fixed patterns in both work and social activities. They have developed firm relationships with co-workers, employees, neighbors, social and recreation associates and others, a status which changes abruptly with the onset of aphasia. Neither the change nor the realization of the degree of change is recognized immediately, but it eventually becomes an important psychosocial consideration in aphasia.

Similarly, aphasics often face an alteration of position in their own family. Again, aphasia most often affects an individual with a major role in a family setting, either as a true leader or as a major contributor to communal activities. If the aphasic disability is comparatively mild, the patient may retain or be able to regain prior status, but when the language disturbance is severe the spouse or some other family member must assume much of the leadership role. Many aphasics find themselves in a passive, child-like position within their own family, needing help from their own children in everyday activities and having most decisions made by their spouse. The aphasic's reaction to this downgrading of position within the family is often violent with negative, hostile, paranoid and downright cruel behavior directed toward close family members. Realization of the alteration of family position is often delayed following the onset of aphasia, and if intelligently and carefully managed the reaction may be minimized. Many families, unfortunately, are not capable of gracefully affecting this alteration. If, instead of offering support, the spouse expresses anger and hostility because of decreased income, altered social position and many new responsibilities, an additional psychological burden is added to the aphasic's troubles. Some deterioration in family position occurs in most aphasic individuals and must be recognized as yet another significant psychological factor.

In addition, many aphasics suffer serious alterations in physical capability. A previously active, self-caring individual may be hemiparetic, must *learn* to stand and walk again and can never again participate in athletic and other physical activities enjoyed in the past. Anyone would be upset by restrictions of this type, and physical impairment is another demoralizing loss to many aphasics.

Still another psychosocial aspect which must be faced eventually by most aphasics is the real or imagined loss of sexual capability. Aphasia-producing pathology does not affect sexual competency in most individuals, but major degrees of paralysis and the inability to communicate accurately create obvious hindrances to normal sexual relationships. Many aphasics suspect that they will never regain sexual prowess, a belief frequently shared by the spouse. In most instances the acquired asexuality is physiologically unnecessary but if both partners believe the condition is real, the normal sexual repsonse may be discouraged. Sexual maladjustment produces additional problems in an aphasic's recovery, one that is almost consistently overlooked by physicians and other therapists.

With the onset of physical illness comes a position of physical incompetence, economic dependence, markedly altered social and employment situations and a decreased stature within the family structure. Because of the many losses, it would be natural for the aphasic to enter into a grief reaction, a period of bereavement. While true grief for an individual physical or social loss may be surmounted, the combination of losses often produces a serious disturbance of self image. With the feeling of self deprecation and worthlessness, a severe depression may result. As a rule, such feelings do not develop immediately but may build over a variable and often extended period after the onset of aphasia.

Against this background it can be anticipated that many aphasic patients will at some stage suffer a period of reactive depression. Actually, while reactive depression does occur in many aphasics, it is far from universal. In fact, the naive observer would anticipate that the disorder of self image should be greater than is apparent in many aphasic patients. Most often this discrepancy reflects the degree of mental deterioration secondary to brain injury rather than the product of an intrinsic ego strength. There are many reasons why reactive depression never becomes a serious problem for many aphasics and these will be discussed later in this chapter. Some aphasic patients, however, do develop a typical reactive depression and suffer intense feelings of personal worthlessness and self-deprecation. The reaction often starts with a sense of futility leading to an unwillingness to participate in rehabilitation measures. During the episode of depression they sink deeply within themselves. They may stop eating, refuse social interaction with therapists, other patients or even family members and show a strong but passive noncooperation. The timing of reactive depression following onset of aphasia is irregular. Aphasics may enter this state soon after onset but more often there is a delay of weeks or even months before the grief reaction sets in.

In general, reactive depression can be considered a healthy sign, indicating sufficient recovery of intellectual competency for recognition of the severity of the problem and the subsequent alterations in life style. From this more realistic status rehabilitation measures can become more problem oriented and the potential for success increases. Nonetheless, reactive depression is an extremely upsetting disturbance for both the patient and those who deal with him. When handled correctly reactive depression in aphasia is usually short-lived but demands careful attention (see Ch. 18).

NEUROBEHAVIORAL ASPECTS

In addition to the psychosocial aspects just outlined, many aphasics suffer alterations of emotional response which appear to vary with the location of pathology within the dominant hemisphere. Correlation of the neuroanatomical loci of pathology with these behavioral changes has only been recognized in recent years. Future studies may produce improved delineation of abnormal anatomical and psysiological influences on the psychological response mechanism but, at present, two behavioral reactions can be correlated with the anatomical locus of pathology. One accompanies selected fluent (posterior) aphasia and the other nonfluent (anterior) aphasia (Benson, 1973).

Most nonfluent aphasics are aware, at least to some degree, of their new problems and tend to become depressed. In addition, the nonfluent aphasic whose output is restricted and effortful often knows exactly what to say but cannot say it, a situation producing intense frustration. Thus, many patients with nonfluent aphasia characteristically experience both depression and frustration. These conditions are potentially serious and, occurring in combination, aggravate each other. If not handled carefully during periods of severe frustration, these patients may develop a serious emotional breakdown that has been called the *catastrophic reaction* (Goldstein, 1948). If nonfluent aphasics are repeatedly asked to perform simple verbal tasks, easily accomplished before the onset of aphasia but now impossible, they can become increasingly frustrated, increasingly depressed and then angry and finally develop an intense emotional breakdown with loud crying, extreme negativity, withdrawal and intense hostility. Patients suffering a fully developed catastrophic reaction stop eating and caring for themselves and arbitrarily refuse communication for days at a time. These patients often refuse to either talk or listen to individuals who previously were of importance, including their own family and members of the hospital staff. Sleep patterns, diet and personal hygiene deteriorate and the patient must be considered dangerously ill. Most catastrophic reactions are short-lived, sometimes lasting only a few hours, but some may continue for a number of days.

The preferred treatment for the catastrophic reaction is prophylactic. The frustrated, depressed, anterior aphasic should never be pushed too hard in language testing. Continual failure is unpleasant for anyone and all the worse for the unfortunate aphasic who knows the correct response but finds that it is locked in. Avoiding humiliation of the aphasic patient is obviously desirable and easily maintained if attention is given to the individual's feelings, not merely the responses given to a test battery. If a catastrophic reaction does take place the major treatment modality is empathy and concern. This, plus the healing course of time, eventually proves successful. Actually, if aphasic patients are handled properly, particularly if not pushed in language testing, the catastrophic reaction will not occur.

Depression in anterior aphasia must always be considered serious. Suicide may be suggested by nonfluent patients and must be accepted as a real possibility. Most anterior aphasics, however, do not represent serious suicidal risks. Early recognition and appropriate alteration of management can prove successful in combatting the depression of anterior aphasia. As an example, a twenty-two-year-old brain-injured soldier with a right hemiplegia and anterior aphasia became acutely depressed when a girlfriend politely but firmly let him understand that she was not interested in marriage to a crippled person. The resulting depression complicated the frustrations of his physical and language disabilities, producing a worrisome situation. Ward personnel were alerted, both to be aware of suicidal potentiality and to offer increased attempts at interrelationships. Therapies were altered to a nonchallenging maintenence level. The process was successful in that the patient recovered from the depths of his grief in only a few days and soon returned to active therapy efforts.

The psychiatric problems noted in patients with fluent (posterior) aphasia are dramatically different. Not only do many individuals with fluent aphasia have problems comprehending spoken language, but they are frequently unaware of their own deficit and in many instances show an abnormal unconcern. The combination of unawareness and unconcern stands in sharp contrast to the frustrated, depressed condition of the anterior aphasic and represents a serious complication. Fluent aphasics, unable to monitor their own verbal output, often fail to realize that their output is incomprehensible jargon. In fact, if a tape recording is made of their jargon and replayed immediately, many will deny that it is their own output. Unaware of their own comprehension disturbance, many posterior aphasics blame their communication difficulties on other individuals. They may suggest that the other individual is not talking clearly enough to be understood or is not paying sufficient attention to what the patient is saying or may even believe that persons they see talking together (but cannot understand) are talking about them in a special code. The tendency to place blame outside the self represents a classic paranoid reaction and may become serious. The paranoia of posterior aphasia is similar, if not identical, to the well-recognized paranoia of acquired deafness. In addition, some posterior aphasics display a tendency for impulsive behavior. The combination of unawareness, paranoia and impulsiveness is serious and makes these patients potentially dangerous, both to themselves and to others. Physical attacks against medical personnel, family members, other patients and themselves can occur. Almost all aphasic patients who need custodial management because of dangerous behavior have a posterior, fluent aphasia (Benson and Geschwind, 1971) with poor comprehension, unawareness of their deficit, paranoia and impulsive behavior. Serious paranoid behavior is particularly common in cases of pure word deafness, less so but still common in Wernicke aphasia, far less common in other posterior aphasias and virtually unknown in anterior aphasia.

Thus, two striking psychiatric responses occur, secondary to specific, anatomically-based aphasic problems, and they occur in addition to the neurobehavioral complications of brain injury discussed in Chapter 16. Combinations of these disorders and the psychosocial factors discussed above are commonplace in aphasia and complicate the total clinical condition immensely.

SUICIDE

A potentially life-threatening psychiatric complication of aphasia, suicide, which may or may not be based on specific neurobehavioral problems, deserves attention. Some aphasic patients do commit suicide and this act must always be considered a serious possibility, particularly in the impulsive posterior aphasic. The depression, frustration and catastrophic reaction of the anterior aphasic would suggest a strong potentiality for suicide, but as already noted, individuals with anterior aphasia rarely even threaten suicide. In caring for over 2,000 aphasics, we have never had an anterior aphasic attempt suicide and few have even suggested that they were thinking of ending their life. Suicide can occur in these patients, however, and reports from other centers document suicide by patients with clear cut anterior aphasia. In our experience suicide is a greater danger in the posterior, fluent aphasic who is both paranoid and impulsive. With increasing awareness of their disability and the profound alterations in life style necessitated by it, the possibility of a premeditated but nonetheless impulsive self-destruction by a posterior aphasic deserves consideration.

The treatment of potential suicide in patients with posterior aphasia is extremely difficult. The inability to communicate freely, based on the comprehension deficit and the incomprehensible jargon output, removes most of the person-to-person (talk-it-out) psychotherapeutic measures currently advised for potential suicide. Standard suicide precautions should be put into effect whenever a suicide wish is suspected, and in addition to the removal of potential self-destructive devices, considerable effort should be made to establish interpersonal relationships and minimize frustration. Even when the suicide potential is recognized and appropriate measures are taken, a well-planned life-ending act can occur. Management of such patients is a tremendous burden that must be shared by all who are in contact with them.

INTELLIGENCE AND LEGAL COMPETENCY

On a totally different level, the physician is often requested to give an expert opinion concerning the mental competency of an aphasic patient, a potentially difficult task. Deciding whether sufficient intelligence is present to warrant investment in long-term rehabilitation therapy itself is often difficult, and determination of legal competency can be almost impossible.

The status of intelligence in aphasia has produced a great deal of disagreement for many years. Following Bastian (1898) who dogmatically stated that "we think in words," many experts have emphasized the symbolic nature of language and the corollary that defective use of symbolization in aphasia produces impaired thinking. On this basis, all individuals with aphasia must have at least some disturbance of intellectual competency. This view reached its zenith with the work of the *gestalt* psychologist Goldstein (1948) who accepted aphasia as a proof of regressed and concrete thinking. Other experts, however, insist that many aphasic patients have comparatively normal intelligence and that it is unjust to place a blanket and derogatory diagnosis of dementia on all. Testing for intelligence in aphasia is made difficult by the inability to use standardized testing procedures, almost all of which rely heavily on verbal instructions and/or responses. Many aphasics perform poorly in both the verbal and nonverbal portions of intelligence tests, suggesting a disturbance of a "general" or underlying factor. Other aphasics, however, show a considerable retention of nonverbal abilities, suggesting considerable residual intelligence. A number of serious studies of intelligence in aphasia have been performed (Tissot, Lhermitte and Ducarne, 1963; Zangwill, 1969; Basso et al, 1973) but at best provide mixed results. Aphasia appears to affect a number of intellectual parameters, but not all. Unfortunately, all psychological studies to date have treated aphasics as a unitary group, not taking into consideration the probability that intellectual deterioration will vary with the syndrome (neuroanatomical locus) of aphasia. It can be suggested that posterior language area pathology is more likely to cause intellectual problems although even this has not yet been systematically demonstrated.

While the presence of aphasia alone may not indicate intellectual loss, there can be no doubt that some aphasic patients suffer combined intellectual and language disturbances. Unfortunately, the contemporary standardized intelligence tests available to most clinicians are not designed to probe this question. Psychologists can provide useful information, particularly by using special test procedures, but most psychometric tests fail to provide unequivocal evidence of the presence or absence of significant intellectual loss in aphasia (see discussion of dementia, Ch. 16). At present, the examiner must base his or her decision on a series of observations. In addition to the results of formal psychological, language and mental status tests, such factors as the retention of social graces, the ability to count and to make change, continued concern about family, business and personal finances, the ability to find one's way about, attempts to socialize with fellow patients, old friends, etc., attention to the immediate environment and appropriate self-concern provide valuable indications of residual intelligence in an aphasic. In general it can be stated that *most aphasics comprehend more than they can indicate and think more clearly than their expressive capability demonstrates.*

Determination of the legal competency of an aphasic may prove severely demanding for the clinician (Critchley, 1970a). Final determination of whether the patient is sufficiently sound mentally to sign checks or business papers, to dispense money, property or other holdings or to make a will often hinges upon informed medical opinion and each aphasic must be judged individually on matters of competency. Many aphasics can manage their own affairs adequately and others are just as obviously unable to make their own decisions and deserve the protection of a conservator or guardian. A third group, however, those who have serious disability, but who with appropriate help can make their own decisions, pose difficult problems and can lead a practitioner into difficult legal controversy. If a legal act (such as signing a will or entering a contract) is to be performed by such an aphasic, the physician should thoroughly evaluate and record the patient's ability to comprehend language and to express personal decisions. Then with the aid of an attorney the document should be reviewed with the patient, bit by bit, until both physician and lawyer are satisfied that the patient understands the basic meaning of the document. This may require several sessions, and for practical reasons the document should be kept as short and simple (free of legalese) as possible.

The most difficult problem of all arises when the practitioner is asked to give retrospective testimony regarding an aphasic patient's legal competency, specifically whether the patient did or did not understand a legal document signed after the onset of aphasia. The physician's testimony can relate only to observations of the patient's mental and language capabilities at or near the time of the signing of the document. The physician's testimony may entail a description of the patient's ability to understand spoken and written language, the ability to express ideas and, if possible, opinion as to mental competency. This is as far as the physician's retrospective testimony should be carried. The final decision will probably depend upon whether the document reflected the patient's wishes at the time of the signing, which is a legal decision, not a medical matter.

In regard to both legal and personal decisions, another general rule can be stated: *aphasic patients should be given the benefit of a great deal of extra effort to allow maintenance of as much control of their own affairs as appears reasonable.* The psychiatric problems in aphasia are often serious but usually not insurmountable, and supportive efforts under the guidance of a concerned clinician will often produce a worthwhile response.

18

Rehabilitation of Aphasia

Until the latter stages of World War II, almost no formal programs for the treatment of aphasia existed. The ensuing years have witnessed a rapid, almost explosive, burgeoning of efforts to rehabilitate the aphasic. Most recorded aphasia therapy prior to WWII was performed by individual neurologists who attempted selected maneuvers on one or a few carefully chosen aphasics, recording and then theorizing about alterations effected. The early formal aphasia therapy efforts lacked specific techniques and featured immense amounts of psychosocial support (sometimes referred to as the "hearts and flowers school of aphasia therapy"). The nonspecificity helped foster a disdain by most practicing neurologists who were well aware that spontaneous improvement occurs in many aphasics and doubted any specific benefit of formal therapy. Until evidence could be provided proving true language benefit from formal language therapy, many practitioners believed that the patient would do as well in the care of the immediate family. With apparent settling of this vexed point (see below), language therapy has branched widely in its search for useful techniques. The subject is changing so rapidly that material presented here will inevitably be dated. Therefore, descriptions of "current" techniques will be brief. This is not to imply that aphasia thereapy is not important; on the contrary, aphasia therapy has already proved valuable in the total rehabilitation of appropriate brain-damaged patients and the future holds considerable promise of increasing help from aphasia therapists.

SPONTANEOUS RECOVERY

Before discussing the techniques utilized for rehabilitation of language loss, the recovery that occurs without treatment deserves consideration. Whether formal therapy is truly effective in improving the outcome of aphasia has long been questioned and many experienced and sincere practitioners still doubt that language therapy exerts any meaningful effect on the recovery of aphasia. Some degree of spontaneous improvement occurs in most aphasics, and cynics maintain that the improvement obtained in aphasia therapy is merely that anticipated from spontaneous recovery. In addition, as Weisenburg and McBride noted (1935), many aphasic patients carry out a program of self training; they respond to their own language problem by developing one or more substitute means of communication.

A number of examiners have investigated the course of spontaneous recovery following onset of aphasia and their observations have been quite consistent (Culton, 1969; Sarno and Levita, 1971; Smith, 1972; Lomas and Kertesz, 1978). In a review of many studies of untreated aphasia Darley (1975) concluded that most spontaneous language recovery occurs in the first month after onset. While improvement may continue for several more months, the amount is so limited that, in his opinion, any significant improvement occurring after this time can be credited to the language therapy. Proof of this observation has been hard to procure.

In recent years, however, the effectiveness of aphasia therapy in overall language recovery has been studied in a more-or-less controlled manner (Basso, Faglioni and Vignolo, 1975; Basso, Capitani and Vignolo, 1979) with clear evidence that as a group aphasics who underwent formal therapy, begun at any stage of recovery, attained better residual language performance than those receiving no formal therapy. Starting with a huge number of aphasics (271), one group received aphasia therapy for at least five months and the other group had no formal therapy. Each patient was tested before and at the end of a six month period with a notable degree of improvement demanded before success could be claimed. A larger number of treated patients improved. The number of patients was sufficiently great that such variables as education, social level, type of aphasia and so forth were matched. The decision for treatment or not was socially determined (whether the patient could travel to the therapy center), however, and this lack of randomization may have permitted some inadvertent bias. The findings from this Italian study, however, strongly suggest that therapy does affect recovery from aphasia. How much of the improvement stems from the psychic support offered by the therapy program and how much is due to actual language training techniques remains unknown. While this study may have technical deficiencies (for the epidemiologist/statistician), it is so large, has sufficiently definite results and would be so difficult to improve upon that it commands respect. It would appear more fruitful to focus future efforts on improving therapy techniques rather than on additional statistical refinements of the treatment-no treatment comparison.

METHODS OF THERAPY

Most therapy currently offered for aphasia can be called "traditional," primarily consisting of techniques of speech training and education, with particular emphasis on rote practice (Darley, 1975). Following initial assessment, the therapist selects the portions of the patient's disability appearing most amenable to available rehabilitation techniques. In an early discussion of recovery from aphasia, Wepman (1951) emphasized three aspects of language therapy: 1) stimulation, an organized presentation of stimuli to procure a reaction; 2) facilitation, repeated practice to increase efficiency at language tasks as they are accomplished and 3) motivation, encouragement for the patient to continue the therapy process. These three approaches continue to represent the bulk of traditional aphasia therapy techniques. At present most aphasia therapy is directed at expressive disturbances, particularly problems of articulation, phonation and the initiation of speech. Reading skills, writing and naming may be treated but therapeutic techniques for improvement of auditory language comprehension are few and have limited success. Fortunately, there is evidence that of all the language functions disturbed in aphasia, comprehension of spoken language is the one most likely to improve spontaneously (Vignolo, 1964).

A number of variations of traditional therapy have been introduced through the years. Weigl (1961, 1968) promoted a formal procedure called *deblocking,* emphasizing the use of intact (or less damaged) language channels to compensate for and actually improve the operation of malfunctioning channels (i.e. presentation of the printed word simultaneously with the spoken word, when one is understood better than the other). Russian therapists (Beyn and Shokhor-Trotskaya, 1966) introduced a technique they called the preventive method to be used in the rehabilitation of patients with expressive language problems. The use of substantive words was curtailed in therapy, emphasizing instead the use of short phrases to avoid development of agrammatic, telegraphic responses during recovery.

Following the introduction of programmed learning techniques in education, programmed therapy was attempted for the aphasic. The original premise that a single well-designed language retraining program could be used for many if not all aphasics was rapidly disproved. Each aphasic is unique and demands an individually designed therapy program, which is an almost unbelievably time-consuming and expensive situation. Nonetheless, many principles of programmed therapy, particularly the technique of repeated practice on the same set of tasks until a consistently successful performance is obtained and then advancing to a more difficult level, are utilized widely in aphasia therapy programs. Traditional therapy for aphasia, then, consists of a mixture of education and speech therapy techniques, often presented in a rigid, "programmed" style.

For many years each aphasic's therapy has been "individually designed"; in other words, the therapist devised a course of therapy based on the presumed needs of the individual patient. While this process sounds both personal and enlightened it often disguises the inadequacies of currently available therapy techniques. In the past few years a number of new therapy techniques have been introduced and it would appear that many more can be expected. The most successful innovation to date has been melodic intonation therapy (MIT) (Sparks, Helm and Albert, 1974). Aphasic patients are taught to tap out the rhythm of a spoken phrase as the phrase is intoned by the therapist, and then while maintaining the rhythmic pattern the patient also attempts to intone the phrase. As intonation becomes successful the therapist gradually withdraws stimulation and the patient can eventually cease rhythm tapping while continuing intonation. Results with MIT have been dramatic in properly selected patients and the technique has rapidly gained world wide use. Careful studies, however, indicate that MIT is useful only for a limited group of aphasics, specifically those with severe output limitations including poor verbal agility, relatively preserved comprehension and poor repetition (essentially Broca aphasia). It has not been successful in Wernicke aphasia or any of the transcortical language disturbances (Helm, 1978).

Another innovation attempts substitution of other means of communication for language. Several recent studies (Eagleson, Vaughn and Knudson, 1970; Chen, 1971) describe the teaching of sign language to the aphasic but report only limited success. Most sign languages (there are a number of varieties) apparently demand as much language competency as spoken language and the ability to use these signs suffers in aphasia. Recent efforts to introduce a one-hand version of Amerind (American Indian) signing have proved considerably more hopeful. Amerind is a communication system, not a language, and appears possible for many aphasics who fail the more complete types of sign language (Skelly et al, 1974). Communication through signing may serve as an additional channel for language stimulation (a channel for deblocking) and thus prove valuable as an adjunct to more traditional aphasia therapy. Even if this does not occur, the learning of a means of communication, even a limited one, may greatly increase the aphasic's ability to interrelate.

On a totally different plane, a variety of machines for communicating have been devised to aid the aphasic. With a few individual exceptions, however, aphasics benefit little from use of the machines. Those aphasics who can master operation of the apparatus almost invariably report easier and better communication without the machine. Almost without exception, aphasics dislike and generally refuse to use machines to aid communication, and the place of electronic gadgetry in the treatment of aphasia remains limited.

Finally, the success of teaching a visual symbol system for communication to chimpanzees (Gardner and Gardner, 1969; Premack, 1971) has stimulated attempts to devise a similar system for use by global aphasics. Preliminary results have not been striking (Glass, Gazzaniga and Premack, 1973; Gardner et al, 1976) but results have been sufficiently encouraging to warrant continued research in this direction (Baker et al, 1976). The most successful symbol communication system reported, visual communication (VIC) (Gardner et al, 1976) utilizes individual 3" × 5" cards, each with a single nonverbal symbol. Through demonstration each card is equated to an object, a person or an action; as "vocabulary" is learned more and more complicated combinations become possible, either for the therapist to present to the patient or vice-versa. Improved verbal language function (both comprehension and naming) has been demonstrated in patients receiving only VIC, and based on this "carryover" a therapy program has been constructed, starting with objects and actions as depicted on cards or by mime and leading to intonation of the appropriate words (Helm and Benson, 1978).

In summary, a number of strikingly different therapy approaches are now being reported and additional innovations can be anticipated. At present, while a specific type of therapy for a specific language deficit is indicated it is not imperative. Traditional therapy is sufficiently broad that it can be molded for use in most aphasic problems. Specific therapy has not been developed for many types of aphasia and thus there is little pressure to select candidates by diagnostic category. MIT, however, has proved effective for a limited group of aphasics and it seems likely that the successful language therapies of the future will be designed for specific language disturbances. Thus, a specific variety of aphasia (e.g. Broca aphasia) will warrant a specific type of therapy. Even without the anticipated advances, it can be stated that many aphasics benefit from aphasia therapy and that almost every aphasic deserves consideration for therapy.

One variety, global aphasia, has consistently proved unrewarding for therapy (Godfrey and Douglass, 1959; Sarno, Silverman and Sands, 1970) and this diagnosis is often considered sufficient grounds in and of itself to withhold therapy. In fact, Schuell and co-workers (1964) were so impressed by this failure that they used the term irreversible for global aphasia and did not recommend therapy. Baker et al (1976), however, have demonstrated that a visual communications system (VIC) could help some global aphasics; additional studies utilizing this and related methods are underway and there is considerable promise for the successful treatment of global aphasia in the future.

Finally, recognition must be given to the important part played by psychic support in aphasia therapy. As noted in Chapter 17, the impairment of language is a cruel blow for the aphasia victim. Employment and economic status are drastically altered and the previous position as family leader, the ability to participate in regular recreational activities and even sexual activities are threatened. Grief, self-concern, frustration and depression frequently complicate the picture of aphasia. Recognition and careful attention to the psychic factors are mandatory for a successful aphasia therapy program.

First the loss, real or threatened, of position in the family is a serious blow, particularly if the individual has been the breadwinner and leader of the family. Careful counseling of the family, helping them to understand the situation and encouraging them to aid the patient in maintaining as much of the prior status as possible is necessary. Altogether too often, however, the family suffers serious problems of their own, some directly attributable to the acute alteration caused by the aphasia but others based on prior difficulties and exacerbated by the patient's condition. Counseling and social support of the family members becomes an essential part of the aphasic's overall therapy program.

Similarly, aphasia is often accompanied by serious physical problems such as hemiplegia, visual disturbance, etc. Full scale rehabilitation programs must be carried out in conjunction with language therapy. Success in a physical rehabilitation program may be reflected by improvement in the language therapy program and vice versa. A well coordinated rehabilitation program includes not only formal physical and language programs but also instruction in the accomplishment of self-care (aids to daily living), recreational therapy and both psychologic and vocational counseling.

The aphasic gets support by working with a person who understands aphasia and is dedicated to the improvement of language deficit. Thus the language therapist as an individual often becomes an important element in the course of recovery. In a similar vein, many aphasics benefit from group interaction. Either observing or actively participating with others who share their disorder appears to offer moral support. Watching other individuals improve and then realizing that they themselves have improved, particularly in comparison to others just entering the program, acts as a source of encouragement for those aphasics capable of appreciating the comparisons. These psychic factors are of importance and they are, at least to some extent, manipulable and deserve attention during aphasia rehabilitation.

Aphasia therapy is a new discipline, one that still remains largely uncharted. Success has been limited to date but the future holds considerable promise. Some future improvements in aphasia therapy may stem from observations currently being made by neurologists, psychologists and linguists working with the aphasic. Others will come from discoveries made by the therapist during training sessions. Yet others, hopefully, will be entirely novel and may well lead to new insights into the mysteries of language for the more academic disciplines.

TREATMENT OF PSYCHIATRIC COMPLICATIONS

In the rehabilitation of any patient, psychological considerations deserve attention. As noted above, great care is needed to be certain that the patient himself, not just the disability, is treated. While most aphasia therapy will be performed by language therapists under the guidance of the patient's physician, problems may arise during rehabilitation that demand neuropsychiatric opinion.

In general, the individual who has lost language ability feels frightened and alone; his ability to cope with everyday problems is diminished and there is a feeling of helplessness. The efforts of a trained therapist, particularly one with experience in the management of aphasia, are appreciated. Not only does the therapist promise expert guidance in the retraining of language function, but the presence of someone who accepts the aphasia, has met it before and is better able to understand and communicate with aphasic patients produces a positive atmosphere. The mere presence of an accomplished therapist acts as a source of psychotherapy. Language therapists, however, have little training in the recognition or management of serious psychiatric problems, and when such problems arise, they may be slow to recognize the difficulty and then may panic, wishing to turn all management of the patient over to a psychiatrist or other physician. This is often a poor solution and in general should be discouraged. As much as possible, a physician should evaluate the patient's condition regularly and counsel the therapist concerning psychiatric problems and measures to alleviate the problem. The experienced language therapist has a better potential for communicating with the aphasic patient; even when the psychiatric problem is serious, demanding active and intense psychiatric management, continued language therapy is often valuable as an additional source of psychotherapy. When the problem is less serious the therapist, under the guidance of the physician or psychiatrist, may be in the best position to offer meaningful psychotherapy. A competent therapist can be a major factor in the successful resolution of most of the psychiatric complications of aphasia.

Reactive depression, as described in Chapter 17, is common and while each patient developing this state deserves close attention, the eventual prognosis is bright. An important factor is early recognition. Hospital personnel and family members dealing with the patient should be alerted regularly to the possibility of a reactive depression and at the first sign of negativism, withdrawal, sleep problems, poor appetite, etc., counter-measures should be undertaken. Reactive depression is a healthy psychic phenomenon in aphasia, and, within limits, it can be allowed to run its course. It is a painful time, however, for both the patient and those about him or her, and demands concern. Extra amounts of sympathy and personal attention (old fashioned tender-loving care) are often rewarded with a rapid recovery. Aphasia therapy should continue during the stage of reactive depression but emphasis should be directed toward positive language features, allowing few failures and many successes rewarded with recognition by the therapist. Eating and sleeping patterns may be altered and medical attention may be needed (such as increased bedtime hypnotic medication), but the problems are most often successfully controlled by intelligent nursing manipulation. While care and attention must be given, the treatment measures should be kept relatively simple. The problem is self-limited and has a basically favorable prognosis; over-treatment may produce unnecessary complications and should be avoided.

The problems of the frustrated, depressed aphasic (see Ch. 17) occasionally demand special management. Continued speech therapy along with a natural tendency for improvement may provide a sufficient boost for morale, but the depression may become sufficiently severe as to interfere with therapy. Recent studies (Folstein, Maiberger and McHugh, 1977; Robinson, 1978) indicate that depression is much more common in cerebral vascular disease than generally realized and suggest that many patients may benefit from appropriate treatment. In our experience antidepressent drugs have not proved highly beneficial for the depressed aphasic but, as they are comparatively safe and simple to administer, they deserve an adequate trial. We have never had to use ECT for the depression of an aphasic but there is no absolute contraindication and ECT can be retained as a possibility if absolutely necessary. Suicide, though admittedly rare, must be kept in mind and proper precautions instituted if necessary (see Ch. 17).

Currently the most effective therapy for the depressed aphasic patient consits of active supportive therapy. This should include ongoing language therapy plus attention to major concerns about family and business obligations. The efforts of a social worker and members of the family, work partners and close friends may be combined to ease the legitimate worries of the depressed aphasic. During the course of rehabilitation, an estimate of the eventual work potential, future financial problems, and necessary alterations in the living arrangements, business responsibilities, etc. should be worked out. Plans should be formulated gradually, with as much participation by the patient as possible. A great deal of support must be given during the period that the patient realizes the limitations on his future. These activities, while usually performed by other members of the rehabilitation team, often need the guidance and direction of the patient's physician.

Involvement in a group often proves useful for the depressed aphasic. The group should be composed entirely of aphasics, preferably individuals with somewhat similar types of aphasia and, to a degree, similar levels of ability. Groups should be supervised by a speech therapist but should feature speech activities, not the self examination or interpersonal criticisms typical of psychiatric groups. Group participation should offer another source of participation, an avenue away from the isolation imposed by the language defect. Some combination of supportive techniques can be instituted and will offer a real "psychotherapy" for the seriously depressed aphasic patient.

Management of the unconcerned, unaware, euphoric and/or paranoid aphasic is totally different. Here the key problem is the patient's unawareness of the language problem, complicated by the inability to communicate with others. When most severe, particularly when a paranoid reaction is present, custodial management, strong tranquilizing medication and continued efforts to establish a means of communication with the patient are indicated. Until the patient develops some awareness of the problem, only the more physical treatments are useful, but with beginning understanding other approaches may prove helpful. Many of these patients appreciate signs and gestures, at least to some degree, and continued attempts to maintain contact by such means are indicated. Language therapy should consist of repeated attempts to communicate with the patient, utilizing spoken, written and/or gestural stimuli. It must be remembered that the limited capacity for the reception and recognition of such stimuli is easily overloaded (Albert and Bear, 1974). Formal therapy requires short, simple stimulations, interspersed with generous rest periods and slow increases in complexity as the patient shows improvement. Similar patterns of slow stimulation and generous rest periods should also be used by the physician and other members of the rehabilitation team when dealing with the patient and, if possible, taught to the family. At least in some situations, the patient's negative reaction toward his own family may stem from their unwitting overloading of the limited capacity to comprehend. Programmed therapy with frequent repetition of the same set of verbal stimuli until the patient is consistently successful and then moving on to a more complicated set of stimuli has proved useful in some instances. The crucial step in therapy for these patients, however, is to obtain realization that there is a real problem, a step over which the therapist has little control. In this early stage, tranquilizers or sedative drugs may be necessary to control aberrant behavior and often appear helpful in the overall therapy program. Whether patients with severe language comprehension problems have auditory hallucinations is unknown but this possibility would not be unacceptable. Possibly control of hallucinations explains the success of the phenothiazines in some cases of posterior aphasia.

Once the patient with posterior aphasia becomes aware of the significant language disability a reactive depression may occur. Supportive management in the manner outlined earlier is indicated but caution must be exercised in choosing the appropriate time to institute supportive management. Until the posterior aphasic realizes that there is a significant language problem, he is a poor candidate for traditional language therapy. To attain this knowledge the patient must be continually impressed with the difficulty. Excessive supportive care offered too early can interfere with this process and can slow recovery. On the other hand, once the problem is realized the patient needs and deserves considerable support.

Finally, a word needs to be included about the management of the mentally ill who develop aphasia. Surprisingly, the added defect may be helpful for the immediate management of preexisting psychiatric disease. Chronic schizophrenics may remain unchanged but individuals with a history of affective illness or episodic psychotic breakdowns rarely show serious exacerbation of mental disability when recuperating from a brain lesion sufficient to cause aphasia. Late in the recovery period, however, return of a prior mental disorder may be seen. Neurotic traits and personality disorders may remain during the acute phases of aphasia but are often so overshadowed by the language disturbance as to require no special attention. Sometimes preexisting mental problems decrease in severity after onset of aphasia and never again demand treatment.

OUTCOME AND RECOVERY

As already intimated in prior sections, variability in the recovery from aphasia is tremendous. Many factors influence the outcome and each patient is quite individual in recovery. Chapter 16 outlines a number of the neurobehavioral disorders frequently seen with aphasia, almost all of which complicate and decrease the capability for recovery. Motivation, probably an organically determined behavioral function, is of obvious significance. In addition to the frequently overlooked neurobehavioral complications, a number of more general factors are also of significance. These include the age at onset, educational level, social status, handedness, etiology and the time elapsed before starting therapy.

The patient's age at the onset of aphasia is a major factor in recovery. In general, the younger the patient, the better the prognosis. Thus individuals who acquire aphasia in childhood have a better chance to recover than middle aged individuals who, in turn, have a better outlook than elderly patients. Many individual exceptions to this rule occur, mostly based on degree and extent of lesion, but it is true to state that, *other factors being equal, the younger the age at the onset of aphasia the better the prognosis.*

Handedness appears to be a significant factor influencing the recovery from aphasia. Luria (1970) noted that left-handed individuals, particularly when young, have a better prognosis for recovery than right-handed individuals.

Whether this is based on a lingering bilaterality for language has not been substantiated but much observational evidence suggests that, *other factors being equal, individuals who are left-handed or ambilateral recover from aphasia faster and more completely than those who are fully right-handed.*

It has been suggested that educational level, social status and socioeconomic background may be significant facotrs in the recovery from aphasia but little absolute evidence supports this statement. It would seem likely that the individual with greater attainments in education and/or higher socioeconomic status would be a better candidate for intensive aphasia therapy. On the other hand, it is far more difficult to rehabilitate a well-educated, professional level individual than a person who has worked at a more physical level. With aphasia, even following good recovery, the attorney, business executive or physician finds it almost impossible to return to prior professional level and such individuals are often reticent to seek employment at a lower level. Returning an aphasic patient to a more manual employment is far easier. This statement does not reflect the degree of recovery from aphasia, however; the professionally trained individual is much more likely to be dependent upon language in his work than the more physically employed person.

There can be no question that the etiology underlying the onset of the aphasia is of immense importance in the recovery process. As a whole, trauma and hematoma cases appear to fare best. The effects of trauma are often widespread, but if there is no residual amnesia the potential for recovery of post-traumatic aphasia is comparatively good. Whether the etiology is a gunshot wound or open or closed head injury, trauma patients on the whole do better than those who suffer occlusive vascular accidents or tumors, possibly because trauma occurs in a younger population. Differences in the long-term prognosis between patients suffering vascular accidents and those with tumor is apparent. The outlook with tumor depends on the course of the disease rather than on the recovery from aphasia. Many intracerebral tumors have a poor prognosis and, therefore, the long-term outcome for the aphasia is of necessity limited. Nevertheless, many patients whose intracerebral tumor has been treated have a life expectancy of several years or more and aphasia therapy can be just as beneficial for them as for patients with other etiologies.

Good evidence suggests that one difference in the degree of recovery from aphasia is based on the time elapsed between the onset of aphasia and the beginning of aphasia therapy (Butfield and Zangwill, 1946; Vignolo, 1964; Darley, 1975). Most accumulated data, however, omit control results on untreated aphasia, and spontaneous improvement is, therefore, included as part of the greater improvement resulting from early initiation of aphasia therapy. There is no proof that commencing aphasia therapy in the first week or even the first month is essential for maximum return of language function. If aphasia therapy is not started until many months or several years after onset, however, the prognosis for significant improvement with aphasia therapy is far more limited. Most aphasia therapists want to see the aphasia patient early and believe that starting therapy within the first few months is highly desirable.

In a masterful review of the pertinent literature plus his own experience in aphasia therapy, Darley (1975) listed nine conclusions concerning the outcome of aphasia therapy: 1) intensive therapy exerts a positive effect on recovery from aphasia; 2) the effects are maximal if therapy is started early and is maintained; 3) the younger the patient the more hopeful the outcome; 4) the underlying etiology affects the outcome of aphasia therapy; 5) milder language losses fare better; 6) better results can be expected if the patient is relatively free of complicating associated disorders; 7) the patient's motivation, insight and other personal factors influence the outcome; 8) no single factor is of such strong negative influence as to preclude at least a trial of therapy; 9) the value of aphasia therapy is not limited to language improvement but also affects attitude, morale and other significant social factors.

In summary, rehabilitation of the aphasic is a relatively new pursuit, a frontier situation both crude and exciting, which already offers valuable assistance to many aphasic patients. The future promises innovative advances in therapy and far greater appreciation of the appropriate technique for a given type of language disturbance. Finally, the statement offered earlier in this chapter bears repetition: *many aphasics benefit from aphasia therapy and almost every aphasic deserves consideration for therapy.*

REFERENCES

Adams, R.D. & Victor, M. (1977). Principles of Neurology. New York: McGraw-Hill.

Adler, A. (1950). Course and outcome of visual agnosia. J. Nerv. Ment. Dis. 3:41–50.

Ajax, E.T. (1967). Dyslexia without agraphia. Arch. Neurol. 17:645–652.

Akelaitis, A.J. (1941). Studies of the corpus callosum II. Arch. Neurol. & Psychiat. 45:788–796.

Akelaitis, A.J. (1944). A study of gnosis, praxis and language following section of the corpus callosum. J. Neurosurg. 1:94–102.

Akelaitis, A.M. (1943). Studies on the corpus callosum, VII-Study of language functions (tactile and visual lexia and graphia) unilaterally following section of the corpus callosum. J. Neuropath. Exptl. Neurology 2:226–262.

Alajouanine, T. (1956). Verbal realization in aphasia. Brain 79:1–25.

Albert, M.L. (1972). Auditory sequencing and left cerebral dominance for language. Neuropsychologia 10:245–248.

Albert, M.L. & Bear, D. (1974). Time to understand. A case study of word deafness with reference to the role of time in auditory comprehension. Brain 97:383–394.

Albert, M.L. & Obler, L.K. (1978). The Bilingual Brain. New York: Academic Press.

Albert, M.L., Sparks, R., Von Stockert, T. & Sax, D. (1972). A case of auditory agnosia: linguistic and non-linguistic processing. Cortex 8:427–443.

Alexander, M.P. & Schmitt, M. (1979). The aphasic syndrome of anterior cerebral artery distribution infarction. Arch. Neurol. (In press).

Alexander, M.P., Stuss, D. & Benson, D.F. (1979). Capgras syndrome. Neurology. (In press).

Alexander, M.P., Stuss, D.T. & Benson, D.F. (1979). Capgras syndrome: a reduplicative phenomenon. Neurology 29:334–339.

Almos-Lau, N., Ginsberg, M.D. & Geller, J.B. (1977). Aphasia in multiple sclerosis. Neurology 27:623–626.

Arendt, H. (1978). The Life of the Mind. New York: Harcourt, Brace Jovanovich.

Baker, E., Berry, T., Gardner, H., Zurif, E., Davis, L. & Veroff, A. (1976). Can linguistic competence be dissociated from natural language functions? Nature 2:609–619.

Barrett, A.M. (1910). A case of pure word-deafness with autopsy. J. Nerv. & Ment. Dis. 37:73–92.

Barton, M., Maruszewski, M. & Urrea, D. (1969). Variation of stimulus context and its effect of word-finding ability in aphasics. Cortex 5:351–365.

Basso, A., Capitani, E. & Vignolo, L.A. (1979). Influence of rehabilitation on language skills in aphasic patients. Arch. Neurol. 36:190–196.

Basso, A., DeRenzi, E. & Fagliani, P. (1973). Neuropsychological evidence for the existence of cerebral areas critical to the performance of intelligence tasks. Brain 96:715–728.

Basso, A., Faglioni, P. & Vignolo, L.A. (1975). Etude contrôlee de la reéducation du langage dans l'aphasie: Comparaison entre aphasiques traités et non-traités. Rev. Neurol. 131:607–614.

Bastian, H.D. (1869). On the various forms of loss of speech in cerebral diseases. Bri. & For. Med. Chic. Rev. 43:209, 470.

Bastian, H.C. (1887). On different kinds of aphasia. Brit. Med. 2:931–936, 985–990.

Bastian, H.C. (1898). Aphasia and Other Speech Defects. London: H.K. Lewis.

Bay, E. (1962). Aphasia and non-verbal disorders of language. Brain 85:411–426.

Bay, E. (1964). Principles of classification and their influence on our concepts of aphasia. In Disorders of Language, eds. De Reuck, A.V.S. & O'Connor, M. Boston: Little, Brown.

Beauvois, M.F., Saillant, B., Meininger, V. & Lhermitte, F. (1978). Bilateral tactile aphasia: A tacto-verbal dysfunction. Brain 101:381–402.

Benson, D.F. (1967) Fluency in aphasia: correlation with radioactive scan localization. Cortex 3:373–394.

Benson, D.F. (1973). Psychiatric aspects of aphasia. Br. J. Psychiat. 123:555–566.

Benson, D.F. (1975). Disorders of Verbal Expression. In Psychiatric Aspects of Neurologic Disorders, eds. Benson, D.F. & Blumer, D. New York: Grune & Stratton.

Benson, D.F. (1977). The third alexia. Arch. Neurol. 34:327–331.

Benson, D.F. (1978). Amnesia. So. Med. J. 71:1221–1227.

Benson, D.F. (1979). Neurologic correlates of anomia. In Studies in Neurolinguistics, Vol. 4, eds. Whitaker, H. & Whitaker, H. (In press).

Benson, D.F. & Blumer, D. (1975). Psychiatric Aspects of Neurologic Disease. New York: Grune & Stratton.

Benson, D.F., Gardner, H. & Meadows, J.C. (1976). Reduplicative paramnesia. Neurology 26:147–151.

Benson, D.F. & Geschwind, N. (1969). The Alexias. In Handbook of Clinical Neurology, Vol. 4, eds. Vinken, P.J. & Bruyn, G.W. Amsterdam: North Holland.

Benson, D.F. & Geschwind, N. (1971). Aphasia and related cortical disturbances. In Clinical Neurology, eds. Baker, A.B. & Baker, L.H. New York: Harper & Row.

Benson, D.F. & Geschwind, N. (1975). Psychiatric conditions associated with focal lesions of the central nervous system. In American Handbook of Psychiatry, Vol. 4, eds. Arietti, S. & Reiser, N. New York: Basic Books.

Benson, D.F., Segarra, J.M. & Albert, M.L. (1974). Visual agnosia-prosopagnosia. Arch. Neurol. 30:307–310.

Benson, D.F., Sheremata, W.A., Buchard, R., Segarra, J., Price, D. & Geschwind, N. (1973). Conduction aphasia. Arch. Neurol. 28:339–346.

Benson, D.F. & Tomlinson, E.B. (1971). Hemiplegic syndrome of the posterior cerebral artery. Stroke 2:559–564.

Benton, A.L. (1961). The fiction of the "Gerstmann Syndrome." J. Neurol. Neurosurg. & Psychiat. 24:176–181.

Benton, A.L. (1964). Contributions to aphasia before Broca. Cortex 1:314–327.

Benton, A.L. (1977). Reflections on the Gerstmann syndrome. Brain & Lang. 4:45–62.

Benton, A.L. & Joynt, R.J. (1960). Early descriptions of aphasia. Arch. Neurol. 3:205–222.

Beyn, E.S. & Shokhor-Trotskaya, M.K. (1966). The preventive method of speech rehabilitation in aphasia. Cortex 2:96–108.

Biemond, A. (1956). The conduction of pain above the level of the thalamus opticus. AMA Arch. Neuro. & Psych. 75:231.

Birkmayer, W. & Neumayer, E. (1972). Rehabilitation of the cerebrovascular patient. In Handbook of Clinical Neurology, Vol. 12, eds. Vinken, P.J. & Bruyn, G.W. Amsterdam: North Holland.

Blumstein, S.E. (1973). A Phonological Investigation of Aphasic Speech. The Hague: Mouton.

Bogen, J.E. (1969). The other side of the brain I: Dysgraphia and dyscopia following cerebral commissurotomy. Bull. LA Neurol. Soc. 34:73–105.

Bogen, J.E. & Bogen, G.M. (1969). The other side of the brain III: The corpus callosum and creativity. Bull. LA Neurol. Soc. 34:191–220.

Boller, F. (1973). Destruction of Wernicke's area without language disturbance. A fresh look at crossed aphasia. Neuropsychologia 11:243–246.

Boller, F., Albert, M.L., LeMay, M. & Kertesz, A. (1972). Enlargement of the sylvian aqueduct: A sequel of head injuries. J. Neurol. Neurosurg. Psychiat. 35:463–467.

Bonvicini, G. (1929). Die storungen der Lautsprache bei Temporallappenläsionen. Handbuch der Neurologie des Ohres. 2:1571–1868. Vienna & Berlin: Urban and Schwarzenberg.

Botez, M.I. & Barbeau, A. (1971). Role of subcortical structures, and particularly of the thalamus, in the mechanism of speech and language. Int. J. Neurol. 8:300–320.

Brain, R. (1941). Visual disorientation with special reference to the lesions of the right cerebral hemisphere. Brain 64:244–272.

Brain, R. (1945). Speech and handedness. Lancet 2:837–842.

Brain, R. (1961). Speech Disorders—Aphasia, Apraxia and Agnosia. London: Butterworth.

Brierley, J.B. (1966). The neuropathology of amnesic states. In Amnesia, eds. Whitty, C.W.M. & Zangwill, O.L. New York: Appleton-Century-Crofts.

Broadbent, D.E. (1971). Decision and Stress. New York: Academic Press.

Broca, P. (1861a). Portée de la parole. Ramollissement chronique et destruction partielle du lobe antérieu gauche du cerveau. Paris Bull. Soc. Anthrop. 2:219.

Broca, P. (1861b). Remarques sur le siège de la faculté du langage articulé, suivies d'une observation d'aphémie. Paris Bull. Soc. Anat. 2:330–357.

Broca, P. (1865). Sur la faculté du langage articulé. Paris Bull. Soc. Anthr. 6:337–393.

Brown, J.R. (1968). A model for central and peripheral behavior in aphasia. Paper delivered at Annual Meeting, Academy of Aphasia, Rochester, Minn.

Brown, J.W. (1972). Aphasia, Apraxia and Agnosia. Springfield, Ill.: Thomas.

Brown, J.W. (1974). Language, cognition and the thalamus. Confin. Neurol. 36:33–60.

Bryden, M.P. (1963). Ear preferences in auditory perception. J. Exp. Psychol. 65:103–105.

Buchwald, L. (1978). Aphasia in progressive multifocal leukodystrophy. Personal communication.

Butfield, E. & Zangwill, O.L. (1946). Re-education in aphasia: a review of 20 cases. J. Neurol. Neurosurg. Psychiat. 9:75–79.

Bychowski, Z. (1919). Ueber die Restitution der nach einem Schädelschuss verlorengegangenen Sprache bei einem Polyglotten. Mtschr. Psychiat. Neurol. 45:184–201.

Campain, R. & Minckler, J. (1976). A note on the gross configurations of the human auditory cortex. Brain & Lang. 3:318–323.

Canter, G. (1971). Observations on neurogenic stuttering: a contribution to differential diagnosis. Br. J. Disord. of Communic. 6:139–143.

Caplan, L. (1972). An investigation of some aspects of stuttering-like speech in adult dysphasic patients. J. So. Afr. Speech Hear Assoc. 19:52–66.

Chapman, L.F. & Wolff, H.G. (1959). The cerebral hemispheres and the highest integrative functions of man. Arch. Neurol. 1:357–424.

Charcot, J.M. (1877). Lectures on the Diseases of the Nervous System. Vol. 1. London: The New Sydenham Society.

Charcot, J.M. (1889). Clinical Lectures on Diseases of the Nervous System. Vol. 3. London: New Sydenham Society.

Chedru, F. & Geschwind, N. (1972). Disorders of higher cortical functions in acute confusional states. Cortex 8:395–411.

Chedru, F., Leblanc, M. & Lhermitte, F. (1973). Visual searching in normal and brain-damaged subjects. Cortex 9:94–111.

Chen, L.C.Y. (1971). Manual communication by combined alphabet and gestures. Arch. Phys. Med. Rehab. 52:381–384.

Chi, J.G., Dooling, E.C. & Gilles, F.H. (1977). Gyral development of the human brain. Annals Neuro. 1:86–93.

Ciemins, V.A. (1970). Localized thalamic hemorrhage: a cause of aphasia. Neurology 20:776–782.

Cole, M. (1968). The anatomical basis of aphasia as seen by Pierre Marie. Cortex 4:172–183.

Conrad, K. (1954). New problems of aphasia. Brain 77:491–509.

Critchley, M. (1930). The anterior cerebral artery and its syndromes. Brain 53:120–165.

Critchley, M. (1952). Articulatory defects in aphasia. J. Laryngol. Otol. 66:1–17.

Critchley, M. (1953). The Parietal Lobes. London: Edward Arnold & Company.

Critchley, M. (1966). The enigma of the Gerstmann's syndrome. Brain 89:183–198.

Critchley, M. (1970a). Testamentary capacity in aphasia. In Aphasiology. London: Edward Arnold Ltd.

Critchley, M. (1970b). Preface to Traumatic Aphasia by A.R. Luria. New York: Basic Books.

Critchley, M. (1970c). Aphasiology. London: Edward Arnold Ltd.

Culton, G.L. (1969). Spontaneous recovery from aphasia. J. Speech Hear. Res. 18:825–832.

Cummings, J., Benson, D.F., Walsh, M.J. & Levine, H. Left to right transfer of language: a case report. Manuscript in preparation.

Cutting, J. (1978). A study of anosognosia. J. Neuro. Neurosurg. Psychiat. 41:548–555.

Darley, F.L. (1968). Apraxia of speech: 101 years of terminological confusion. Unpublished paper presented at annual meeting, American Speech and Hearing Association.

Darley, F.L. (1975). Treatment of acquired aphasia. In Advances in Neurology. Vol. 7, ed. Friedlander, W.J. New York: Raven Press.

Darley, F.L. Aronson, A.E. & Brown, J.R. (1969). Differential diagnostic patterns of dysarthria. J. Speech Hear. Res. 12:246–269.

Darley, F.L. Aronson, A.E. & Brown, J.R. (1975). Motor Speech Disorders. Philadelphia: Saunders.

Dax, M. (1836). Lésions de la moitié gauche de l'encéphale coincident avec trouble des signes de la pensie. Paper presented in Montpelier.

Dejerine, J. (1891). Sur un cas de cécité verbale avec agraphie, suivi d'autopsie. Mem. Soc. Biol.. 3:197–201.

Dejerine, J. (1892). Contribution à l'étude anatomo-pathologique et clinique des différentes variétés de cécité verbale. Mem. Soc. Biol. 4:61–90.

DeMasio, A.R. & Kassel, N.F. (1978). Transcortical motor aphasia in relation to lesions of the supplementary motor area. Presentation to 30th annual meeting, American Academy of Neurology, Los Angeles, Cal.

DeRenzi, E., Faglioni, P. & Scotti, G. (1970). Hemispheric contribution to exploration of space through the visual and tactile modality. Cortex 6:191–203.

DeRenzi, E. Pieczuro, A. & Vignolo, L.A. (1966). Oral apraxia and aphasia. Cortex 2:50–73.

DeRenzi, E., & Vignolo, L.A. (1962). The token test: A sensitive test to detect receptive disturbances in aphasics. Brain 85:665–678.

Dubois, J., Hecaen, H. & Marcie, P. (1969). L'agraphie "pure". Neuropsychologia 7:271–286.

Dubois, J., Mazars, G., Marcie, P. & Hecaen, H. (1966). Étude des performances aux épreuves linguistiques des sujets atteints de syndromes parkinsoniens. L'Encéphale 55:496–513.

Eagleson, H.M., Vaughn, G.R. & Knudson, A.B. (1970). Hand signals for dysphasia. Arch. Phys. Med. & Rehab. 51:111–113.

Eisenson, J. (1954). Examining for Aphasia. New York: Psychological Corp.

Farmakides, M.N. & Boone, D.R. (1960). Speech problems of patients with multiple sclerosis. J. Speech Hear. Disorder 25:385–390.

Fedio, P. & Van Buren, J.M. (1975). Memory and perceptual deficits during electrical stimulation in the left and right thalamus and parietal subcortex. Brain & Lang. 2:78–100.

Fischer, C.M. (1975). The anatomy and pathology of the cerebral vasculature. In Modern Concepts of Cerebrovascular Disease, ed. Meyer, J.S. New York: Spectrum.

Folstein, M.F., Maiberger, R. & McHugh, P.R. (1977). Mood disorder as a specific complication of stroke. J. Neuro. Neurosurg. Psychiat. 40:1018–1020.

Freud, S. (1891, 1953). On Aphasia. Trans. E. Stengl. New York: Int. Univ. Press.

Freund, C.S. (1888). Ueber optische Aphasie und Seelenblindheit. Arch. Psychiat. Nervenkhr. 20:276–297.

Gainotti, G. (1972). Emotional behavior and hemispheric side of the lesion. Cortex 8:41–55

Gainotti, G. Messerli, P. & Tissot, R. (1972). Qualitative analysis of unilateral spatial neglect in relationship to laterality of cerebral lesions. J. Neuro. Neurosurg. Psychiat. 35:45–550.

Galaburda, A.M., LeMay, M., Kemper, T.L. & Geschwind, N. (1978). Right-left asymmetries in the brain. Science 199:852–856.

Galin, D. (1974). Implications for psychiatry of left and right cerebral specialization. Arch. Genl. Psych. 31:572–583.

Gardner, H. (1973). The contribution of operativity to naming capacity in aphasic patients. Neuropsychologia 11:213–220.

Gardner, H., Zurif, E., Berry, T. & Baker, E. (1976). Visual communication in aphasia. Neuropsychologia 14:275–292.

Gardner, R.A. & Gardner, B. (1969). Teaching sign-language to a chimpanzee. Science 165:664–672.

Gazzaniga, M.S. (1970). The Bisected Brain. New York: Appleton-Century-Crofts.

Gazzaniga, M.S., Glass, A.A., Sarno, M.T. & Posner, J.B. (1973). Pure word deafness and hemispheric dynamics: a case history. Cortex 9:136–143.

Gazzaniga, M.S. & Sperry, R.W. (1967). Language after section of the cerebral commissures. Brain 90:131–148.

Gerstmann, J. (1931). Zur Symptomatologie der Hirnläsionen im Uebergangsgebiet der unteren Parietal-und mittleren Occipitalwindung. Nervenarzt. 3:691–695.

Geschwind, N. (1965). Disconnexion syndromes in animals and man. Brain 88:237–294, 585–644.

Geschwind, N. (1967a). The Apraxias. Proceedings of the Second Lexington VAH Conference on Will and Action, eds. Strauss & Griffith. Duquesne University Press.

Geschwind, N. (1967b). The varieties of naming errors. Cortex 3:97–112.

Geschwind, N. (1967c). Wernicke's contribution to the study of aphasia. Cortex 3:449–463.

Geschwind, N. (1977). Psychiatric Complications in the Epilepsies: Introduction McLean Hospital Journal, June 1977, pp. 6–8.

Geschwind, N. & Fusillo, M. (1966). Color naming defects in association with alexia. Arch. Neurol. 15:137–146.

Geschwind, N. & Kaplan, E.F. (1962). A human cerebral deconnection syndrome. Neurology, 12:675–685.

Geschwind, N. & Levitsky, W. (1968). Human brain: left-right asymmetries in temporal speech region. Science 161:186–187.

Geschwind, N., Quadfasel, F.A. & Segarra, J. (1968). Isolation of the speech area. Neuropsychologia 6:327–340.

Glass, A.V., Gazzaniga, M.S. & Premack, D. (1973). Artificial language training in global aphasias. Neuropsychologia 11:95–103.

Gloning, K. (1977). Handedness and aphasia. Neuropsychologia 15:355–358.

Gloning, I., Gloning, K., Haub, C. & Quatember, R. (1969). Comparison of verbal behavior in right-handed and non right-handed patients with anatomically verified lesion of one hemisphere. Cortex 5:43–52.

Gloning, I., Gloning, K. & Hoff, H. (1963). Aphasia—a clinical syndrome. In Problems of Dynamic Neurology. ed Halpern, L. Jerusalem: Hebrew University.

Gloning, I., Gloning, K., Seitelberger, F. & Tschabitscher, H. (1955). Ein Fall von reiner Wortblindheit mit Obduktionsbefund. Wien Z. Nervenheilk 12:194–215.

Godfrey, C. & Douglass, E. (1959). The recovery process in aphasia. Canad. Med. Assoc. J. 80:618–624.

Goldstein, K. (1917). Die Transkortikalen Aphasien. Jena, Gustav Fischer.

Goldstein, K. (1924). Das Wesen der amnestischen Aphasie. Schweiz. Arch. f. Neurol. und Psychiat. 15:163–175.

Goldstein, K. (1948). Language and Language Disturbances. New York: Grune & Stratton.

Goldstein, M. (1974). Auditory agnosia for speech (pure word deafness): A historical review with current implications. Brain & Language 1:195–204.

Goldstein, M., Joynt, R. & Goldblatt, D. (1971). Word blindness. Neurology 21:873–876.

Goldstein, M.N., Brown, M. & Hollander, J. (1975). Auditory agnosia and cortical deafness: analysis of a case with three years follow-up. Br. & Lang. 2:324–332.

Goodglass, H. & Baker, E. (1976). Semantic field naming and auditory comprehension in aphasia. Br. & Lang. 3:359–374.

Goodglass, H., Barton, M.I. & Kaplan, E. (1968). Sensory modality and object-naming in aphasia. J. Speech & Hearing Res. 11:488–496.

Goodglass, H. & Berko, J. (1960). Agrammatism and inflectional morphology in English. J. Speech & Hearing Res. 3:257–267.

Goodglass, H. & Blumstein, S. (1973). Psycholinguistics and Aphasia. Baltimore: Johns Hopkins.

Goodglass, H., Gleason, J.B., Bernholtz, N.A. & Hyde, MR (1972). Some linguistic structures in the speech of a Broca's aphasic. Cortex 8:191–212.

Goodglass, H. & Kaplan, E. (1972). The Assessment of Aphasia and Related Disorders. Philadelphia: Lea & Febiger.

Goodglass, H. & Quadfasel, F. (1954). Language laterality in left handed aphasics. Brain 77:521–548.

Goodglass, H., Quadfasel, F. & Timberlake, W. (1964). Phrase length and the type and severity of aphasia. Cortex 1:133–153.

Green, E. & Howes, D. (1977). Conduction aphasia. In Studies in Neurolinguistics. Vol. 3, eds. Whitaker, H. & Whitaker, H.A. New York: Academic Press.

Greenblatt, S.H. (1973). Alexia without agraphia or hemianopsia. Brain 96:307–316.

Greenblatt, S.H. (1976). Subangular alexia without agraphia or hemianopsia. Brain & Language 3:229–245.

Greenblatt, S. (1977). Neurosurgery and the anatomy of reading: A practical review. Neurosurgery 1:6–15.

Guttman, E. (1942). Aphasia in children. Brain 65:205–219.

Haase, G.R. (1977). Diseases presenting as dementia. In Dementia-Edition 2, ed. Wells, C.E. Philadephia: Davis.

Hachinski, V.C., Lassen, N.A. & Marshall, J. (1974). Multi-infarct dementia: a cause of mental deterioration in the elderly. Lancet 3:207–210.

Head, H. (1926). Aphasia and Kindred Disorders (2 volumes). London: Cambridge University Press.

Hecaen, H. (1962). Clinical symptomatology in right and left hemisphere lesions. In Interhemispheric Relations and Cerebral Dominance, ed. Mountcastle, V.B. Baltimore: Johns Hopkins.

Hecaen, H. (1969). Essai de dissociation du syndrome de l'aphasie sensorielle. Rev. Neurol. 120:229–231.

Hecaen, H. (1976). Acquired aphasia in children and the ontogenesis of hemispheric functional specialization. Brain & Language 3:114–134.

Hecaen, H. & Albert, M.L. (1978). Human Neuropsychology. New York: Wiley.

Hecaen, H. & Angelerques, R. (1964). Localization of symptoms in aphasia. In Disorders of Language, eds. DeReuck, A.V.S. & O'Conner, M. London: Churchill.

Hecaen, H. & Angelergues, R. (1965). Pathologie du Langage. Paris: Larousse.

Hecaen, H., Angelergues, R. & Douzenis, J.A. (1965). Les agraphies. Neuropsychologia 3:217–247.

Hecaen, H. & Consoli, S. (1973). Analyse des troubles du langage au cours des lésions de l'aire de Broca. Neuropsychologia 11:377–388.

Hecaen, H., Dell, M.B. & Roger, A. (1955). L'aphasie de conduction. L'Encéphale 2:170–195.

Hecaen, H. & Marcie, P. (1974). Disorders of written language following right hemisphere lesions: spatial dysgraphia. In Hemispheric Function in the Human Brain, eds. Dimond, S.J. & Beaumont, J.G. London: Elek. Science.

Heilman, K. (1973). Ideational apraxia—a re-definition. Brain 96:861–864.

Heilman, K. (1979). Apraxia. In Neurobehavioral Problems, ed. Heilman, K. London: Oxford. (In press.)

Heilman, K.M. & Valenstein, E. (1972). Auditory neglect in man. Arch. Neurol. 26:32–35.

Heilman, K.M., Watson, R.T. & Schulman, H.M. (1974). A unilateral memory defect. J. Neurol. Neurosurg. Psychiat. 37:790–793.

Heimburger, R.F., Demyer, W. & Reitan, R.M. (1961). Implications of Gerstmann's syndrome. J. Neurol. Neurosurg. Psychiat. 27:53–57.

Helm, N.A. (1978). Criteria for selecting aphasic patients for melodic intonation therapy. Presented to annual meeting of AAAS, Washington, D.C.

Helm, N. & Benson, D.F. (1978). Visual action therapy for global aphasia. Presentation, 16th Annual Meeting, Academy of Aphasia, Chicago, Ill.

Helm, N.A., Butler, R.B. & Benson, D.F. (1978). Acquired stuttering. Neurology 28:1159–1165.

Helm, N.A. & Leiberman, A. (1977). Management of palilalia with a pacing board. Presented to annual meeting, American Speech and Hearing Assoc., Chicago, Ill.

Henneberg, R. (1918). Reine Worttaubheit. Neur. zbl. 37:426–427

Henschen, S.E. (1922). Klinische und Anatomische Beitrage zur Pathologie des Gehirns. Stockholm: Almquist and Wiksell.

Hier, D.B., Davis, K.R., Richardson, E.P. & Mohr, J.P. (1977). Hypertensive putaminal hemorrhage. Annals Neuro. 1:152–159.

Hier, D.B. & Mohr, J.P. (1977). Incongruous oral and written naming: Evidence for a subdivision of the syndromes of Wernicke aphasia. Brain & Lang. 4:115–126.

Hinshelwood, J. (1900). Letter-Word and Mind-Blindness. London: H.K. Lewis.

Holland, A.L. (1977). Assessment of Communicative Activities Relevant to Daily Living. Research project sponsored by NIH.

Holmes, G. (1918). Disturbances of vision by cerebral lesions. Brit. J. Ophth. 2:353–384.

Hoops, R. & Lebrun, Y., eds. (1974). Intelligence and Aphasia. Amsterdam: Swetts & Zeitlinger, B.V.

Horel, J.A. (1978). The neuroanatomy of amnesia: a critique of the hippocampal memory hypothesis. Brain 101:403–445.

Howes, D. (1964). Application of the word frequency concept to aphasia. In Disorders of Language, eds. DeReuk, A.V.S. & O'Connor, M. London: Churchill.

Howes, D. & Boller, F. (1978). Comparison of lesion size in radioisotope brain scan with actual pathology at post-mortem. Personal communication.

Howes, D. & Geschwind, N. (1964). Quantitative studies of aphasic language. In Disorders of Communication Proc. ARNMD, Baltimore: Williams & Wilkins.

Ingvar, D.H. & Schwartz, M.D. (1974). Blood flow patterns induced in the dominant hemisphere by speech and reading. Brain 97:274–288.

Isserlin, M. (1929). Die pathologische Physiologie der Sprache. Ergebn. Physiol. 29:129–149.

Isserlin, M. (1931). Die pathologische Physiologie der Sprache. Ergebn. Physiol. 33:1–102.

Isserlin, M. (1932). Die pathologische Physiologie der Sprache. Ergebn. Physiol. 34:1065–1144.

Jackson, J.H. (1864). Clinical remarks on cases of defects of expression (by words, writing, sighs, etc.) in diseases of the nervous system. Lancet 1:604–605.

Jackson, J.H. (1932). Selected writings, ed. Taylor. London: Hodder & Stoughton.

Jakobson, R. (1964). Towards a linguistic typology of aphasic impairments. In Disorders of Language, eds. DeReuck, A.V.S. & O'Connor, M. Boston: Little, Brown.

Johns, D.F. & Darley, F.L. (1970). Phonemic variability in apraxia of speech. J. Speech Hearing Res. 13:556–583.

Karis, R. & Horenstein, S. (1976). Localization of speech parameters by brain scan. Neurology 26:3:226–231.

Katz, J.J. & Foder, J.A. (1964). The structure of a semantic theory. Language 29:170–

210. Reprinted in Katz, J.A. and Forder, J.J. eds. The Structure of Language. Englewood Cliffs, N.J.: Prentice-Hall.

Kennard, M. (1939). Alterations in response to visual stimuli following lesions of the frontal lobe in monkeys. Arch. Neurol. & Psychiat. 41:1153–1165.

Kennedy, F. & Wolf, A. (1936). The relationship of intellect to speech defect in aphasic patients. J. Nerv. & Ment. Dis. 84:125–145, 293–311.

Kertesz, A. & Benson, D.F. (1970). Neologistic jargon—a clinico-pathological study. Cortex 6:362–386.

Kertesz, A., Lesk, D. & McCabe, P. (1977). Isotope localization of infarcts in aphasia. Arch. Neurol. 34:590–601.

Kertesz, A. & McCabe, P. (1977). Recovery patterns and prognosis in aphasia. Brain 100:1–18.

Kertesz, A. & Phipps, J.B. (1977). Numerical taxonomy of aphasia. Br. & Lang. 4:1–10.

Kertesz, A. & Poole, E. (1974). The aphasia quotient: the taxonomic approach to measurement of aphasic disability. Canad. J. Neurol. Sciences 1:7–16.

Kimura, D. (1967). Functional asymmetry of the brain in dichotic listening. Cortex 3:163–178.

Kinsbourne, M. & Rosenfield, D.B. (1974). Agraphia selective for written spelling. Br. & Lang. 1:215–226.

Kinsbourne, M. & Warrington, E.K. (1962). A variety of reading disability associated with right hemisphere lesions. J. Neurol. Neurosurg. Psychiat. 25:339–344.

Klein, R. & Harper, J. (1956). The problem of agnosia in the light of a case of pure word deafness. J. Ment. Sci. 102:112–120.

Kleist, K. (1934a). Gehirnpathologie. Leipzig: Barth.

Kleist, K. (1934b). Leitungsaphasie (Nachsprechaphasie). In Handbuch der Aertzlichen Erfahrungen im Weltkriege 1914/1918, ed. Bonhoeffer, K. Leipzig: Barth.

Kløve, H., Grabow, J.D. & Trites, R.L. (1969). Evaluation of memory functions with intracarotid sodium amytal. Trans. Am. Neurol. Assoc. 94:76–80.

Krashen, S. (1973). Lateralization, language learning and the critical period. Lang. Learning 23:63–74.

Kremer, M., Russell, W.R. & Smyth, G.E. (1947). A mid-brain syndrome following head injury. J. Neuro. Neurosurg. & Psychiat. 10:49–60.

Kurtzke, J.F. (1970). Clinical manifestations of multiple sclerosis. In Handbook of Clinical Neurology Vol. 9, eds. Vinken, P.J. & Bruyn, G.W. Amsterdam: North Holland.

Lambert, W. & Fillenbaum, S. (1959). A pilot study of aphasia among bilinguals. Canad. Journ. of Psychol. 13:28–34.

Landau, W.M., Goldstein, R. & Kleffner, F.R. (1960). Congenital aphasia: a clinico-pathologic study. Neurology 10:915–921.

Larsen, B., Skinhøj, E. & Endo, H. (1977). Localization of basic speech functions as revealed by 12 CBF measurements in normals and in patients with aphasia.In Cerebral Vascular Disease 8th Int. Salzburg Conference, eds. Meyer, A.S., Lechner, M. & Revich, M. Amsterdam: Excerpta Medica.

Larsen, B., Skinhøg, E. & Lassen, N.A. (1978). Variations in regional cortical blood flow in the right and left hemispheres during automatic speech. Brain 101:193–210.

Lashley, K.S. (1926). Studies of cerebral function in learning VII: the relation between cerebral mass, learning and retention. J. Comp. Neurol. 41:1–58.

Lashley, K.S. (1929). Brain Mechanisms and Intelligence. Chicago: University of Chicago Press.

LeCours, A.R. & Lhermitte, F. (1969). Phonemic paraphasias: linguistic structures and tenative hypotheses. Cortex 5:193–228.

Lehman, J.R., DeLateur, B.J. & Fowler, R.F., Jr. (1975). Does rehabilitation affect outcome? Arch. Phys. Med. Rehab. 56:383–389.

Leischner, A. (1957). Die störungen der Schriftsprache (Agraphie und Alexie). Stuttgart: Georg Thieme Verlag.

LeMay, M. & Culebras, A. (1972). Human brain-morphologic differences in the hemispheres demonstrable by carotid angiography. NEJM 287:168–170.

Lenneberg, E. (1967). Biological Foundations of Language. New York: Wiley.

Levin, H.S., Grossman, R.G. (1978). Behavioral sequelae of closed head injury. Arch. Neurol. 35:712–719.

Levine, D.N. (1978). Prosopagnosia and visual object agnosia: A behavioral study. Br. & Lang. 5:341–365.

Lhermitte, F. & Beauvois, M.F. (1973). A visual-speech disconnexion syndrome. Brain 96:695–714.

Lhermitte, F., Chain, F. & Escourelle, R. (1972). Etude anatomo-clinique d'un cas de prosopagnosie. Rev. Neurol. 126:329–346.

Lhermitte, F. & Gautier, J.C. (1969). Aphasia. In Handbook of Clinical Neurology, Vol. 4, eds. Vinken, P.J. & Bruyn, G.W. Amsterdam: North Holland.

Lichtheim, L. (1885). On aphasia. Brain 7:433–484.

Lieberman, A. & Benson, D.F. (1977). Pseudobulbar palsy. Arch. Neuro. 34:717–719.

Liepmann, H. (1900). Das Krankheitsbild der Apraxie ('motorischen Asymbolie'). Berlin: Karger.

Liepmann, H. (1905). Das Krankheitsbild der Apraxie. Mschr. Psychiat. Neurol. 17:289–311.

Liepmann, H. & Storck, E. (1902). Ein Fall von reiner Sprachtaubheit. Mschr. Psychiat. Neurol. 11:225.

Lipowski, Z.J. (1975). Organic brain syndrome: overview and classification. In Psychiatric Aspects of Neurologic Disease, eds. Benson, D.F. & Blumer, D. New York: Grune & Stratton.

Lishman, A.W. (1978). Organic Psychiatry. Oxford: Blackwell.

Lomas, J. & Kertesz, A. (1978). Patterns of spontaneous recovery in aphasic groups: a study of adult stroke patients. Br. & Lang. 5:388–401.

Lombroso, C.T. & Erba, G. (1970). Primary and secondary bilateral synchrony in epilepsy. Arch. Neurol. 22:321–334.

Luria, A.R. (1964). Neuropsychology in the local diagnosis of brain damage. Cortex 1:3–18.

Luria, A.R. (1966). Higher Cortical Functions in Man. New York: Basic Books.

Luria, A.R. (1970). Traumatic Aphasia. The Hague: Mouton.

Luria, A.R. (1977). On quasi-aphasic speech disturbances in lesions of the deep structures of the brain. Br. & Lang. 4:432–459.

Marie, P. (1906a). Révision de la question de l'aphasie. Semaine Med. 26:241–247.

Marie, P. (1906b). Révision de la question de l'aphasie. Semaine Med. 26:493–500.

Marie, P. (1906c). Révision de la question de l'aphasie. Semaine Med. 26:565–571.

Marie, P. & Foix, C. (1917). Les aphasies de guerre. Rev. Neurol. 24:53–87.

Martin, J.P. (1954). Pure word blindness considered as a disturbance of visual space perception. Proc. Roy. Soc. Med. 47:293–295.

Maruszewski, M. (1975). Language, Communication and the Brain. The Hague: Mouton.

Maspes, P.E. (1948). Le syndrome expérimental chez l'homme de la section du splenium corps calleux, alexie visuelle pure hémianopsique. Revue Neurologie 2:101–113.

McRae, D.L., Branch, C.L. & Milner, B. (1968). The occipital horns and cerebral dominance. Neurology 18:95–98.

Merleau-Ponty, M. (1964). Signs. Evanston: Northwestern U Press.

Meyer, J.S., Sakai, F., Nautenu, H. & Grant, P. (1978). Normal and abnormal patterns of cerebrovascular reserve tested by 133 Xe inhalation. Arch. Neurol. 35:350–359.

Milner, B. (1974). Hemispheric specialization: Scope and limits. In The Neurosciences Third Study Program, eds. Schmitt, F.O. & Worden, F.G., Cambridge: MIT.

Milner, B., Branch, C. & Rasmussen, T. (1964). Observations on cerebral dominance. In Disorders of Language, eds. DeReuk, A.V.S. & O'Connor, M. London: Churchill.

Mohr, J.P. (1973). Rapid amelioration of motor aphasia. Arch. Neurology 28:77–82.

Mohr, J.P., Finkelstein, S., Pessin, M.S., Duncan, G.W. & Davis, K. (1975). Broca's area infarction versus Broca's aphasia. Presentation to 27th Annual Meeting of American Academy of Neurology, Bal Harbor, Florida, May 7th.

Mohr, J.P., Pessin, M.S., Finkelstein, S., Funkenstein, H.H., Duncan, G.W. & Davis, K.R. (1978). Broca aphasia: pathologic and clinical aspects. Neurology 28:311–324.

Mohr, J.P., Watters, W.C. & Duncan, G.W. (1975). Thalamic hemorrhage and aphasia. Br. & Lang. 2:3–17.

Monrad-Krohn, G.H. (1947). Dysprosody of altered melody of language. Brain 70:405–415.

Muller, R. (1949). Studies in disseminated sclerosis with special reference to symptomatology. Acta Med. Scand. Suppl. 222.

Naeser, M.A. & Hayward, R.W. (1978). Lesion localization in aphasia with cranial computed tomography and the Boston Diagnostic Aphasia Exam. Neurology 28:545–551.

Nathan, P.W. (1947). Facial apraxias and apraxic dysarthria. Brain 70:449–478.

Nielsen, J.M. (1936, 1962). Agnosia, Apraxia and Aphasia. Their Value in Cerebral Localization. New York: Hafner.

Nielsen, J.M. (1938). The unsolved problems in aphasia: I. Alexia in "motor" aphasia. Bull. LA Neurol. Soc. 4:114–122.

Nielsen, J.M. (1939). The unsolved problems in aphasia: II. Alexia resulting from a temporal lesion. LA Neurol. Soc. 5:78–84.

Nielsen, J.M. (1940). The unsolved problems in aphasia: Part III. Amnesic Aphasia. Bull. LA Neurol. Soc. 5:78–84.

Obler, L.K. & Albert, M.L. (1977). Influence of aging on recovery from aphasia in polyglots. Br. & Lang. 4:460–463.

Obler, L.K., Albert, M.L., Goodglass, H. & Benson, D.F. (1978). Aphasia type and aging. Br. & Lang. 5:318–322.

Ojemann, G. & Ward, A. (1971). Speech representation in ventrolateral thalamus. Brain 94:669–680.

Oppenheimer, D.R. & Newcombe, F. (1978). Clinical and anatomical findings in a case of auditory agnosia. Arch. Neurol. 35:706–711.

Orgass, B., Hartje, W., Kerschensteiner, M. & Poeck, K. (1972). Aphasie und nichtsprachliche intelligenz. Nervenarzt 43:623–627.

Osgood, C.E., Suci, G.J. & Tannenbaum, P.H. (1957). The Measurement of Meaning. Urbana, Ill.: U. of Ill. Press.

Oxbury, J.M., Campbell, D.C. & Oxbury, S.M. (1974). Unilateral spatial neglect and impairments of spatial analysis and visual perception. Brain 97:551–565.

Paradis, M. (1972). Bilingualism and aphasia. In Studies in Neurolinguistics, Vol. 3, eds. Whitaker, H. and Whitaker, H. New York: Academic Press.

Penfield, W. & Roberts, L. (1959). Speech and Brain Mechanisms. Princeton: Princeton University Press.

Pick, A. (1913). Die Agrammatischen Sprachstorungen. Berlin: Springer.

Pick, A. (1931, 1973). Aphasia. Springfield, Ill.: Charles C. Thomas.

Piercy, M. (1964). The effects of cerebral lesions on intellectual function. Br. J. Psychiat. 110:310–352.

Pincus, J.H. & Tucker, G. (1974). Behavioral Neurology. New York: Oxford.

Pitres, A. (1895). Etude sur l'aphasie chez les polyglottes. Rev. Med. 15:873–899.

Poeck, K. (1972). Stimmung und Krankheitseinsicht bei Aphasien. Arch. Psychiat. Nervenkr. 216:246–254.

Poeck, K., Kerschensteiner, M. & Hartje, W. (1972). A qualitative study on language understanding in fluent and non-fluent aphasia. Cortex 8:299–304.

Poeck, K. & Orgass, B. (1969). An experimental investigation of finger agnosia. Neurology 19:501–507.

Popper, K.R. & Eccles, J.C. (1977). The Self and its Brain. New York: Springer.

Porch, B. (1967). Porch Index of Communicative Ability. Palo Alto: Consulting Psychologists.

Posner, C.M. (1975). Personal communication.

Premack, O. (1971). Language in the chimpanzee. Science 172:808–822.

Quadfasel, F.A. (1968). Aspects of the life and work of Kurt Goldstein. Cortex 4:113–124.

Ravens, J.C. (1952). Human Nature: Its Development, Variations and Assessment. London: H.K. Lewis.

Ribot, T. (1883). Les Maladies de la Mémoire. Paris: Libraire Germer Bailliere.

Riklan, M. & Levita, E. (1970). Psychological studies of thalamic lesions in humans. J. Nerv. Ment. Dis. 150:251–265.

Ring, B.A. (1969). The Neglected Cause of Stroke. St. Louis: W.H. Green.

Ring, B.A. & Waddington, M.M. (1968). Occlusion of small intracranial arteries as a cause of stroke. JAMA 204:303–305.

Roberts, L. (1969). The relationship of cerebral dominance to hand, auditory and ophthalmic preference. In Handbook of Clinical Neurology, Vol. 4, eds. Vinken, P.J. & Bruyn, G.W. Amsterdam: North Holland.

Robinson, R.G. (1978). Affect/Mood Scale. Unpublished research questionnaire.

Rochford, G. & Williams, M. (1962). Studies in the development and breakdown of the use of names. I: The relationship between nominal dysphasia and the acquisition of vocabulary in childhood. J. Neurol. Neurosurg. Psychiat. 25:222–227.

Rochford, G. & Williams, M. (1965). Studies in the development and breakdown of the use of names. IV: The effects of word frequency. J. Neurol. Neurosurg. Psychiat. 28:407–413.

Romanul, F.C.A. (1970). Examination of the Brain and Spinal Cord. In Neuropathology, ed. Tedeschi, C.G. Boston: Little, Brown.

Romanul, F.C.A. & Abramowitz, A. (1961). Changes in brain and pial vessels in arterial borderzones. Arch. Neurol. 11:40–49.

Rosenbek, J., Messert, B., Collins, M. & Wertz, R.T. (1978). Stuttering following brain damage. Br. & Lang. 6:82–96.

Rosenfield, D.B. & Goree, J.A. (1975). Angiographic localization of aphasia. Neurology 35:349.

Rubens, A.B. (1976). Transcortical motor aphasia. In Studies in Neurolinguistics, Vol. I, eds. Whitaker, H. & Whitaker, H.A. New York: Academic Press.

Rubens, A.B. (1977). The role of changes within the central nervous system during recovery from aphasia. In Rationale for Adult Aphasia Therapy, Proceedings of a Conference held at the University of Nebraska Medical Center, eds. Sullivan, M. & Kommers, M. U. of Nebraska Medical Center.

Rubens, A.B. & Benson, D.F. (1971). Associative visual agnosia. Arch. Neurol. 24:305–315.

Russell, W.R. & Espir, M.L.E. (1961). Traumatic Aphasia—A Study of Aphasia in War Wounds of the Brain. London: Oxford University Press.

Rutter, D.R., Draffan, J. & Davies, J. (1977). Thought disorder and the predictability of schizophrenic speech. Br. J. Psychiat. 131:67–68.

Sahs, A.L. & Hartman, E. (1976). Fundamentals of Stroke Care. DHEW Publ. No(HRA) 76–14016.

Sak, K., Larsen, B., Shinhøj, E. & Lassen, N.A. (1978). Regional cerebral blood flow in aphasia. Arch. Neurol. 35:625–632.

Samarel, A., Wright, T.L., Sergay, S. & Tyler, H.R. (1976). Thalamic hemorrhage with speech disorder. Trans. Am. Neuro. Ass. 101:283–285.

Samuels, J. & Benson, D.F. (1979). Observations on anterior alexia. Br. & Lang. (In press.)

Sarno, M.T. & Levita, E. (1971). Natural course of recovery in severe aphasia. Arch. Phys. Med. Rehab. 52:175–178.

Sarno, M.T. & Sands, E. (1970). An objective method for the evaluation of speech therapy in aphasia. Arch. Phys. Med. Rehab. 52:49–54.

Sarno, M.T., Silverman, M. & Sands, E. (1970). Speech therapy and language recovery in severe aphasia. J. Speech Hear. Res. 13:607–623.

Sasanuma, S. (1975). Kana and Kanji processing in Japanese aphasics. Br. & Lang. 2:369–383.

Sasanuma, S. & Fujimura, O. (1971). Kanji versus Kana processing in alexia with transient agraphia: a case report. Cortex 7:1–18.

Schiller, F. (1947). Aphasia studied in patients with missile wounds. J. Neuro. Neurosurg. & Psychiat. 10:183–197.

Schmitt, (1948). Pure word deafness. (Quoted by Goldstein, K. in Language & Language Disturbances.) New York: Grune & Stratton.

Schuell, H. (1957). Minnesota Test for the Differential Diagnosis of Aphasia. Minneapolis: University of Minnesota Press.

Schuell H., Jenkins, J.J. & Jimenez-Pabon, E. (1964). Aphasia in Adults—Diagnosis, Prognosis and Treatment. New York: Hoeber.

Schuster, P. & Taterka, H. (1926). Beitrag zur Anatomie und Klinik der reinen Worttaubheit. Zschr. f.d. ges Neur. U. Psychiat. 105:494–538.

Schwab, O. (1926). Ueber vorubergehende aphasische störungen nach Rindenexzision aus dem linken stirnhirn bei Epileptikern. Dtsche Zschr. Nervenhlk 94:177–184.

Segarra, J.M. (1970). Cerebral vascular disease and behavior. Arch. Neurol. 22:408–418.

Serafatinides, E.A. (1966). Auditory recall and visual recognition following intracarotid amytal. Cortex 2:367–372.

Shankweiler, D. & Studdert-Kennedy, M. (1967). Identification of consonants and vowels presented to the left and right ears. Quant. J. Exp. Psychol. 19:59–63.

Simernitskaya, E.G. (1974). On two forms of writing defect following local brain lesions. In Hemispheric Function in the Human Brain, eds. Dimond, S.J. & Beaumont, J.G. London: Elek Science.

Skelly, M., Schinsky, L., Smith, R.W. & Fust, R.S. (1974). American Indian sign (Amerind) as a facilitator of verbalization for the oral verbal apraxic. JSHD 39:445–456.

Sklar, M. (1966). Sklar Aphasia Scale. Los Angeles: Western Psychological Services.

Smith, A. (1966). Speech and other functions after left dominant hemispherectomy. J. Neurol. Neurosurg. Psychiat. 29:467–471.

Smith, A. (1972). Diagnosis, Intelligence and Rehabilitation of Chronic Aphasics: Final Report. Ann Arbor: University of Michigan.

Smith, A. & Sugar, O. (1975). Development of above-normal language and intelligence 21 years after left hemispherectomy. Neurology 25:813–818.

Souques, A. (1928). Quelques cas d'anarthrie de Pierre Marie. Rev. Neurolog. 2:319–368.

Sparks, R. & Geschwind, N. (1968). Dichotic listening in man after section of neocortical commissures. Cortex 4:3–16.

Sparks, R., Goodglass, H. & Nickel, B. (1970). Ipsilateral versus contralateral extinction in dichotic listening from hemispheric lesions. Cortex 6:249–260.

Sparks, R., Helm, N. & Albert, M. (1974). Aphasia rehabilitation resulting from melodic intonation therapy. Cortex 10:303–316.

Spellacy, F. (1970). Lateral preferences in the identification of patterned stimuli. J. Acoust. Soc. Amer. 47:574–578.

Sperry, R.W. & Gazzaniga, M.S. (1967). Language following surgical disconnection of the hemispheres. In Brain Mechanisms Underlying Speech and Language, ed. Darley, F.L. New York: Grune & Stratton.

Spreen, O. & Benton, A. (1960). Neurosensory Center Comprehensive Examination for Aphasia. Victoria: Neuropsychology Laboratory, University of Victoria.

Spreen, O., Benton, A. & Fincham, R. (1965). Auditory agnosia without aphasia. Arch. Neurol. 13:84–92.

Spreen, O., Benton, A.L. & Van Allen, M.W. (1966). Dissociation of visual and tactile naming in amnesic aphasia. Neurology 16:807–814.

Stengel, E. (1947). A clinical and psychological study of echo reactions. J. Ment. Sci. 93:598–612.

Strub, R.L. & Gardner, H. (1974). The repetition deficit in conduction aphasia: amnestic or linguistic? Br. & Lang. 1:241–256.

Taylor, M.L. (1968). A measurement of functional communication in aphasia. Arch. Phys. Med. Rehab. 46:101–107.

Taylor, W.L. (1953). 'Cloze Procedure': a new tool for measuring readability. Journalism Quart. 30:415–433.

Teuber, H.L. (1968). Alteration of perception and memory in man. In Analysis of Behavioral Change, ed. Weizkrantz, L. New York: Harper & Row.

Tissot, R., Lhermitte, F. & Ducarne, B. (1963). Etat intellectuel des aphasiques. Essai d'une nouvelle approche à travers des épreuves perceptives et opératoires. Le'Encéphale 52:285–320.

Trescher, J.H. & Ford, F.R. (1937). Colloid cyst of the third ventricle. Arch. Neurol. & Psyc. 37:959–973.

Trost, J. (1971). Apraxic dysfluency in patients with Broca's aphasia. Presented at annual meeting, American Speech and Hearing Assoc., Chicago, Ill.

Trost, J.E. & Canter, G.L. (1974). Apraxia of speech in patients with Broca's aphasia. Br. & Lang. 1:63–79.

Trousseau, A. (1864). De l'aphasie, maladie décrite récemment sans le nom impropre d'aphémie. Gaz. Hop (Paris) 37:13, 25, 37, 49.

Tzortzis, C. & Albert, M.L. (1974). Impairment of memory for sequences in conduction aphasia. Neuropsychologia 12:355–366.

Van Buren, J.M. (1975). The question of thalamic participation in speech mechanisms. Br. & Lang. 2:31–44.

Van Buren, J.M. & Burke, R.C. (1969). Alterations in speech and the pulvinar. Brain 92:255–284.

Victor, M., Adams, R.D. & Collins, G.H. (1971). The Wernicke-Korsakoff Syndrome. Philadelphia: F.A. Davis.

Vignolo, L. (1964). Evolution of aphasia and language rehabilitation: a retrospective exploratory study. Cortex 1:344–367.

Vignolo, L.A. (1969). Auditory agnosia: A review and report of recent evidence. In Contributions to Clinical Neuropsychology, ed. Benton, A.L. Chicago: Aldine.

Von Monakow, C. (1914). Die Lokalisation im Grosshirn und der Abbau der Funktion durch korticale Herde. Wiesbaden: Bergmann.

Von Monakow, C. & Bourque, R. (1928). Introduction Biologique à l'étude de la Neurologie et de la Psychiatrie. Paris: Alcan.

Wada, J. & Rasmussen, T. (1960). Intracarotid injection of sodium amytal for the lateralization of cerebral speech dominance: experimental and clinical observations. J. Neurosurg. 17:266–282.

Wagenaar, E., Snow, C. & Prins, R. (1975). Spontaneous speech of aphasic patients: a psycholinguistic analysis. Br. & Lang. 2:281–303.

Warrington, E.K. (1969). Constructional apraxia. In Handbook of Clinical Neurology, Vol. 4, eds. Vinken, P.J. & Bruyn, G.W. Amsterdam: North Holland.

Warrington, E.K. & Shallice, T. (1969). The selective impairment of auditory verbal short-term memory. Brain 92:885–896.

Watson, R.T. & Heilman, K.M. (1978). Thalamic neglect. Presented at the Annual Meeting, American Academcy of Neurology, Los Angeles.

Wechsler, I. (1952). Textbook of Clinical Neurology, 7th Ed. Philadelphia: Saunders.

Weigl, E. (1961). The phenomenon of temporary deblocking in aphasia. Z.f. Phon. Spr. u. Komm 14:337–364.

Weigl, E. (1968). On the Problem of Cortical Syndromes. In The Reach of Mind: Essays in Memory of Kurt Goldstein, ed. Simmel, M.L. New York: Springer.

Weisenburg, T.S. & McBride, K.L. (1935, 1964). Aphasia. New York: Hafner.

Weinstein, E.A. & Cole, M. (1963). Concepts of anosognosia. In Problems of Dynamic Neurology, ed. Halpern, L. Jerusalem: Hebrew Univ.

Weinstein, E.A. & Kahn, R.L. (1952). Non-aphasic mixnaming (paraphasia) in organic brain disease. Arch. Neurol. & Psychiat. 67:72–79.

Weinstein, E.A. & Kahn, R.L. (1955). Denial of Illness: Symbolic and Physiologic Aspects. Springfield, Ill.: Charles C. Thomas.

Weinstein, E.A. & Keller, N.J.A. (1973). Linguistic patterns of misnaming in brain injury. Neuropsychologia 1:79–90.

Wells, C.E. (1977). Dementia—2nd Edition. Philadelphia: Davis.

Wepman, J. (1961). Language Modalities Test for Aphasia. Chicago: Education Industry Service.

Wepman, J.M. (1951). Recovery from Aphasia. New York: Ronald.

Wepman, J.M. & Jones, L.V. (1964). Five aphasias: A commentary on aphasia as a regressive linguistic problem. In Disorders of Communication ARNMD, 42. Baltimore: Williams & Wilkins.

Wernicke, K. (1874). Der Aphasische Symptomkomplex. Breslau: Kohn & Neigart.

Wernicke, K. (1881). Lehrbuch der Gehirnkrankheiten. Berlin: Theodor Fischer.

Wernicke, K. (1908). The symptom complex of aphasia. In Modern Clinical Medicine: Diseases of the Nervous System, ed. Church, E.D. New York: Appleton-Century-Crofts.

Whitaker, H. (1976). A case of the isolation of the language function. In Studies in Neurolinguistics, Vol. 2, eds. Whitaker, H. & Whitaker, H. New York: Academic Press.

Whitaker, H. & Whitaker, H.A. (1976a). Studies in Neurolinguistics, Vol. 1. New York: Academic Press.

Whitaker, H. & Whitaker, H.A. (1976b). Studies in Neurolinguistics, Vol. 2. New York: Academic Press.

Whitaker, H. & Whitaker, H.A. (1976b). Studies in Neurolinguistics, Vol. 3. New York: Academic Press.

Whitaker, H. & Whitaker, H.A. (1979). Studies in Neurolinguistics, Vol. 4. New York: Academic Press.

Whitty, C.W.M. (1964). Cortical dysarthria and dysprosody of speech. J. Neurol. Neurosurg. Psychiat. 27:507–510.

Wildmore, L.J., Wilder, B.J., Mayersdorf, A., Ramsay, R.E. & Sypert, G.W. (1978). Identification of speech lateralization by intracarotid injection of methohexital. Annals Neuro. 4:86–88.

Wilson, S.A.K. (1926). Aphasia. London: Kegal Paul.

Wylie, J. (1894). The Disorders of Speech. Edinburgh: Oliver and Boyd.

Yakovlev, P.I. & Rakic, P. (1966). Patterns of decussation of bulbar pyramids and distribution of pyramidal tracts on two sides of the spinal cord. Trans. Amer. Neurol. Assoc. 91:366–367.

Yamadori, A. (1975). Ideogram reading in alexia. Brain 98:231–238.

Yarnell, P., Monroe, M.A. & Sobel, L. (1976). Aphasia outcome in stroke: a clinical and neurological correlation. Stroke 7:516–522.

Zangwill, O.L. (1960). Cerebral Dominance and its Relation to Psychological Function. Springfield, Ill.: Charles C. Thomas.

Zangwill, O.L. (1969). Intellectual status in aphasia. In Handbook of Clinical Neurology, Vol. 4, eds. Vinken, P.J. & Bruyn, G.W. Amsterdam: North Holland.

Ziehl, F. (1896). Ueber einen Fall von Worttaubheit und das Lichtheim'sche krankheitsbild der subcorticalen sensorischen Aphasie. Deutsche ztschr. f. Nervenheilkunde 8:259–307.

Zurif, E.B., Caramazza, A. & Myerson, R. (1972). Grammatical judgments of agrammatic aphasics. Neuropsychologia 10:405–417.

Index